ALZHEIMER'S DIAGNOSIS

NEUROSCIENCE RESEARCH PROGRESS

Additional books in this series can be found on Nova's website
under the Series tab.

Additional E-books in this series can be found on Nova's website
under the E-books tab.

ALZHEIMER'S DIAGNOSIS

CHARLES E. RONSON
EDITOR

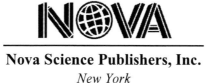

Nova Science Publishers, Inc.
New York

Library of Congress Cataloging-in-Publication Data

Alzheimer's diagnosis / editor, Charles E. Ronson.
   p. ; cm.
  Includes bibliographical references and index.
  ISBN 978-1-61209-846-3 (hardcover)
  1. Alzheimer's disease--Diagnosis. I. Ronson, Charles E.
  [DNLM: 1. Alzheimer Disease--diagnosis. WT 155]
  RC523.A36756 2011
  616.8'31--dc22
                2011004496

Published by Nova Science Publishers, Inc. † New York

Contents

Preface

The demographics of aging suggest a great need for an early diagnosis of dementia and for the development of preventive strategies. Neurodegeneration in Alzheimer's disease is estimated to start 20-30 years before clinical onset, and the identification of biological markers for pre-clinical and early diagnosis is the principal aim of research studies in the field. In this book, the authors present topical research on Alzheimer's diagnosis including cerebrospinal fluid biomarker Amyloid-B 1-42 identification; visual impairment in Alzheimer's disease; cerebral glucose metabolism through F-fluoro-deoxy-glucose positron emission tomography and neuroimaging. (Imprint: Nova Biomedical Press)

Chapter I - Today, the diagnosis of Alzheimer's disease (AD) is based on the identification of symptoms like dementia and other clinical indications. Cerebrospinal fluid (CSF) biomarkers like the level of amyloid-β 1-42 (Aβ42), which is lower in AD patients than in controls, or the levels of total Tau and phosphorylated Tau, which are enhanced, are supposed to increase the diagnostic accuracy or might even be valuable for earlier diagnosis. However, the monomeric form of Aβ is not thought to be responsible for neurotoxocity and neurodegeneration. Aβ monomers are non-pathogenic metabolic products also abundant in healthy humans. Aβ oligomers were identified as the most toxic species in AD which arise early in the disease progress and the amount of Aβ oligomers in the brain correlates well with cognitive impairment. Therefore, presence of Aβ oligomers can be expected to be a more direct disease biomarker for AD and increasing effort is being made into the development of methods suitable for the detection of different Aβ aggregates in body fluids like CSF and plasma. Here, we review the current status of assay development to reliably and routinely detect Aβ oligomers in body fluids. Additionally, we compare the outcomes of the different assay systems.

Chapter II - Alzheimer's Disease (AD) is the most common cause of dementia in the older adults world-wide. About 4.5 million individuals in USA currently are estimated to be affected and by mid-century the prevalence will be 11.3-16 million cases (Cronin-Golomb and Hof, 2004). AD is viewed as a disorder primarily of memory, that represents usually the initial sign; moreover, this disease is characterized by impairment in several additional domains, including visual function. However, the NINCDS-ADRDA clinical diagnostic criteria (Tierney et al., 1988) make no mention of sensory changes. Several main fields of researches on vision in AD currently are undertaken, from structure to function and behavior at this time, and current directions in AD vision studies are extensively reported in many papers, including some exhaustive books (Cronin-Golomb and Hof, 2004). In summary, this chapter spans the visual impairment in AD patients, from structure to function, either at retinal or cortical levels in an attempt to highlight visual sub-system changes, particularly the magnocellular, in AD compared to normal aging and other age-related degenerative disorders.

Chapter III - Clinical neuroscience has an increasing need for new methods to identify the earliest features of neurodegenerative disorders such as Alzheimer's disease (AD) and other dementias. This growing interest in the pre-dementia phase of these conditions aims to identify them before functional impairment is evident. Ideally before this phase, treatment of the underlying disease would postpone its process. A variety of clinical, imaging and laboratory methods has emerged during the last decade to allow more accurate diagnosis of AD. A review of these new markers will be made with reference to the new diagnostic criteria proposed by the International Working Group in Alzheimer's disease.

Chapter IV - The relations between Japanese Alzheimer's disease (AD) patients and their mitochondrial single nucleotide polymorphism (mtSNP) frequencies at individual mtDNA positions of the entire mitochondrial genome were examined using the radial basis function (RBF) network and the modified method. Japanese AD patients were associated with the haplogroups G2a, B4c1, and N9b1. In addition, to compare mitochondrial haplogroups of the AD patients with those of other classes of Japanese people, the relations between four classes of Japanese people (i.e., Japanese centenarians, Parkinson's disease (PD) patients, type 2 diabetic (T2D) patients, and non-obese young males) and their mtSNPs were also analyzed by the proposed method. The four classes of people were associated with following haplogroups: Japanese centenarians—M7b2, D4b2a, and B5b; Japanese PD patients—M7b2, B4e, and B5b; Japanese T2D patients—B5b, M8a1, G, D4, and F1; and Japanese healthy non-obese young males— D4g and D4b1b. The haplogroups of the AD patients are therefore different from those of other four classes of Japanese people. As the analysis method described in this article can predict a person's mtSNP constitution and the probabilities of becoming an AD patient, centenarian, PD patient, or T2D patient, it may be useful in initial diagnosis of various diseases.

Chapter V - Early detection of Alzheimer's disease (AD) is particularly important to reveal preclinical pathological alterations, to monitor disease progression and to evaluate treatment response. The study of cerebral glucose metabolism through ^{18}F-fluoro-deoxy-glucose positron emission tomography (FDG-PET) plays a leading role in early detection of AD because the decrease of cerebral glucose metabolism largely precedes the onset of AD symptoms. This technique demonstrated high sensitivity in early diagnosis of AD allowing a qualitative and quantitative estimate of cerebral glucose metabolism. Furthermore FDG-PET imaging may help discriminate the subjects who more probably could develop AD in a high-risk population (as patients with mild cognitive impairment). A limit of FDG-PET is the lack of specificity; in fact the decrease of cerebral glucose metabolism is a common feature of various dementias. Nevertheless AD patients generally show hypometabolism of medial temporal lobes and parieto-temporal posterior cortices in early stage; other cortices are involved in more advanced AD stages. The combination of FDG-PET with other biomarkers such as genotype, cerebrospinal fluid markers and tracers for amyloid plaque imaging may increase the preclinical diagnostic accuracy and offer promising approaches to assess individual prognosis in AD patients.

Chapter VI - A clear tendency of an aging population (2.5 billion elders are estimated on a global scale by the year 2050) has brought about an increase of its associated diseases, one of which is the higher prevalence dementia focusing in *Alzheimer's Disease* (AD). Today, it is estimated that there are 18 million people suffering from AD worldwide, and the disease affects 5% -10% of 65-year old and more than 30% of 85-year old. This situation has important repercussions in the scope of the patient but also in the familiar, social and sanitary spheres. Therefore, early diagnosis of AD is a major public healthcare concern, and the *Differential Diagnosis of Dementia* (DDD) is also one of the crucial points to which clinical medicine faces at every level of attention. The definite diagnosis of AD is only post-mortem. Furthermore, there are not yet a specific set of diagnostic criteria for the confirmation of the diagnosis. In this context it's necessary to develop new alternative methods and instruments of diagnosis, especially on early and differential diagnosis, and introducing its use in all healthcare areas. This chapter will be dedicated to explore the ability of a complementary approach to face these problems, the Artificial Neural Networks (ANNs). The ANNs are highly non-linear systems. Its more appealing property is its learning capability. Its behaviour emerges from structural changes driven by local learning rules, having the capability of generalisation. In addition to this approach, especially computer-intensive algorithms based on "ensemble learning"-methods that generate many classifiers and aggregate their results are being developed in regard of Mild Cognitive Impairment (MCI), AD and DDD classification. We will present a study of ANNs, where it will be analysed a new neural architecture, HUMANN-S, which has shown to be a very suitable ANN for Alzheimer's diagnosis scope. The neural network ensemble approach is introduced. Finally we will discuss the ability of ANN and neural network ensembles, to address this issue, describing the outcomes of implementations of such approaches for AD, DDD and MCI diagnosis using for the inputs several types of data: Electroencephalogram (EEG) type signals, neuroimages, like Single Photon Emission Computerized Tomography (SPECT), and/or scores of different neuropsychological tests, among others.

Chapter VII – Progressive aging of population will make Alzheimer's Disease (AD) one of the most important health problems of the next years, challenging social security and health systems of industrialized countries. The present work analyzes the resources and the difficulties of the diagnostic flow charts in territorial reality where more important space is given to the clinical activity rather than to research. When first symptoms of a possible dementia appear, people contact general practioner, directly or pushed by their relatives. The general practioner is very important for the screening in case of a possible dementia because his/her attention and sensibility make early diagnosis possible. General practioner, in fact, usually requires a consult to the specialist (neurologist, psychiatric, geriatrician), which, working in équipe with the psychologist, can begin a multi-dimentional evaluation of first level that includes: 1) medical history; 2) general and neurological examination; 3) neuropsychological screening; 4) evaluation of functional abilities; 5) assessment of patient's relationship and family context; 6) routine and specific blood tests; 7) at least one neuroimaging exam (e.g. CT scan). Undoubtedly, the results of the clinical and instrumental investigations may provide useful elements for the differential diagnosis of dementia and, therefore, for adequate medical, psychological and socio-relational caring. However, the diagnostic process remains, to date, a puzzle that clinicians build progressively due to the lack of specific biomarkers.

Chapter VIII - The demographics of aging suggest a great need for an early diagnosis of dementia and for the development of preventive strategies. Neurodegeneration in Alzheimer's disease (AD) is estimated to start even 20–30 years before clinical onset, and the identification of biological markers for pre-clinical and early diagnosis is the principal aim of research studies in the field. It is still difficult to make diagnosis in the early disease stages. At the beginning the patient might have a deficit limited to memory or to another single cognitive domain, without any disorder of instrumental and daily activities. The cognitive impairment then might proceed to a degree that allows the diagnosis of dementia. The transitional state between normal ageing and mild dementia has been recently indicated by the term Mild Cognitive Impairment (MCI). In the last few years, a wide range of studies addressed this topic. Clinically, within the group of MCI subjects, two separate subgroups have been described, those rapidly converting to AD (MCI converters), in whom MCI represents the early stage of an ongoing AD-related process, and those who remain stable (MCI non-converters), in whom the isolated cognitive deficits represent a different condition without an increased risk to develop dementia at short follow-up. In this line, reliable markers for early AD detection could be useful both for prognosis, and for identifying a potential target for therapeutic intervention, since treatments are emerging which rather than reversing structural damage are likely to slow or halt the disease process. While currently no routine diagnostic test confirms AD presence, functional neuroimaging techniques represent an important tool in biological neurology. The challenge for neuroimaging methods is to achieve high specificity and sensitivity in early disease stages and at single subject level. Functional imaging, in particular, has the potential to detect very early brain dysfunction even before clear-cut neuropsychological deficits emerge. Predicting progression to AD in cases of MCI and supporting diagnosis and differential diagnosis of dementia are the outmost important goals. The implications are the identification of minimally symptomatic patients that could benefit from treatment strategies, as well as the monitoring of treatment response and the therapeutic deceleration of the disease. This chapter highlights recent cross-sectional and longitudinal neuroimaging studies in the attempt to put into perspective their value in diagnosing AD-like changes, particularly at an early stage, providing diagnostic and prognostic specificity. There is now considerable evidence supporting that early diagnosis is feasible through a multimodal approach, including also a combination of multiple imaging modalities.

Chapter IX - Alzheimer's disease (AD), Lewy-body disease (LBD) and Frontotemporal Dementia (FTD) are the major causes of memory impairment and dementia. As new therapeutic agents are under testing for the different diseases, there is an ultimate need for an early differential diagnosis. Biomarkers can serve as early diagnostic indicators or as markers of preclinical pathological changes. Therefore, diagnostic markers in the cerebrospinal fluid (CSF) have become a rapidly growing research field, since CSF is in direct contact with the central nervous system (CNS) and is supposed to reflect the brain environment. So far, three CSF biomarkers, the 42 amino acid form of β-amyloid (Aβ), total tau and phosphotau, have been validated in a number of studies. These CSF markers have high sensitivity to differentiate early and incipient AD from normal aging, depression, alcohol dementia and Parkinson's disease, but lower specificity against other dementias, such as FTD and LBD. This chapter reviews CSF biomarkers for AD, with emphasis on their role in the clinical diagnosis.

In: Alzheimer's Diagnosis
Editor: Charles E. Ronson, pp. 1-24

ISBN: 978-1-61209-846-3
©2011 Nova Science Publishers, Inc.

Chapter I

Quantitation of Amyloid-B Oligomers in Human Body Fluids for Alzheimer's Disease: Early Diagnosis or Therapy Monitoring?

Susanne Aileen Funke and Dieter Willbold

Institute of Complex Systems (ICS-6),
Forschungszentrum Jülich, Jülich, Germany
Institut für Physikalische Biologie, Heinrich-Heine-Universität,
Düsseldorf, Germany

Abstract

Today, the diagnosis of Alzheimer's disease (AD) is based on the identification of symptoms like dementia and other clinical indications. Cerebrospinal fluid (CSF) biomarkers like the level of amyloid-β 1-42 (Aβ42), which is lower in AD patients than in controls, or the levels of total Tau and phosphorylated Tau, which are enhanced, are supposed to increase the diagnostic accuracy or might even be valuable for earlier diagnosis.

However, the monomeric form of Aβ is not thought to be responsible for neurotoxocity and neurodegeneration. Aβ monomers are non-pathogenic metabolic products also abundant in healthy humans. Aβ oligomers were identified as the most toxic species in AD which arise early in the disease progress and the amount of Aβ oligomers in the brain correlates well with cognitive impairment.

Therefore, presence of Aβ oligomers can be expected to be a more direct disease biomarker for AD and increasing effort is being made into the development of methods suitable for the detection of different Aβ aggregates in body fluids like CSF and plasma.

Here, we review the current status of assay development to reliably and routinely detect Aβ oligomers in body fluids. Additionally, we compare the outcomes of the different assay systems.

Introduction

Alzheimer's disease (AD) is a devastating neurodegenerative disorder and the most common cause of dementia, which accounts for 60 to 80 percent of the estimated cases. The clinical characteristics are difficulties remembering names and recent events, apathy and depression at the beginning, later followed by impaired judegment, disorientation, confusion, behavior changes and difficulties in speaking, swallowing and walking. The greatest risk factor for AD is advancing age (aged 65 or older), but most scientists agree that AD is not a normal part of aging (Alzheimer's association). AD affects 27 million people world-wide (1) with steadily increasing tendency, thereby raising significant personal and economic problems.

Currently, the only definite diagnosis of AD is the post mortem detection of amyloid plaques and neurofibrillary tangles in the brain tissue of the deceased patient. Diagnosis of AD during lifetime is based on the identification of the symptoms described above and physiological screening tests for cognitive impairment like the Mini-Mental Status Examination (MMSE) or the Alzheimer's Disease Assessment Scale (2, 3).

Even in specialized centers it is challenging to diagnose AD at early stages, and diagnosis based on clinical symptoms will always fail to reveal presymptomatic cases. The sensitivity and specificity of clinical diagnosis for AD is 70 to 80 percent only in specialized centers and even lower for patients with early AD or in primary care settings (4-6). Several publications support the finding that plaques and tangles start to accumulate 10 to 20 years before the symptoms appear, leading to substantial neuronal loss (7-9).

Therefore, the challenge is to diagnose individuals at earlier stages, when the disease is still presymptomatic and perhaps more amenable to treatment. At present, only symptomatic treatment of AD is available, but several compounds are currently being developed, most of them aiming at Aβ, e.g. secretase inhibitors, immunotherapy and Aβ aggregation inhibitors (10, 11). More than 10 compounds are currently in clinical phase III trials, and much more in phases I or II (Alzforum). Referring to PubMed, hundreds of compounds are in the preclinical state.

One of the biggest obstacles for AD therapy development is the lack of biomarkers which reflect the core pathology of AD and the disease state and progression, not dependent of clinical symptoms as they arise late in AD pathology and are difficult to detect adequately.

One biomarker probably suited to fulfill the requirements is the amyloid-β (Aβ) peptide. Aβ is the major component of the amyloid plaques. It consists of 39 to 43 amino acid residues. Aβ, especially Aβ42, is prone to aggregation and undergoes formation from monomers to oligomers, larger intermediate forms like protofibrils, insoluble fibrils and plaques (12). Aβ is derived from the amyloid precursor protein (APP) by sequential activities of the β- and γ-secretases (13-15). As originally suggested by the amyloid cascade hypothesis (16), it appears likely that Aβ peptides and their aggregated forms initiate cellular events leading to the pathologic effects of AD. According to a prevoius version of the amyloid cascade hypothesis, fibrillar forms of Aβ in amyloid plaques have been thought to be responsible for neuronal dysfunction (16, 17). More recent studies support that diffusable Aβ oligomers, including protofibrils, prefibrillar aggregates and so called Aβ-derived diffusible ligands (ADDLs), are the major toxic species during disease development and progression (18-21).

More or less validated clinical methods for the determination of Aβ load in vivo are the visualization of the amyloid plaque load in the living brain using amyloid-binding tracers like Pittsburgh Compound B (PIB) in positron emission tomography (PET) (22) or the detection of monomeric Aβ in the cerebrospinal fluid (CSF) via ELISA or ELISA-like methods (23, 24).

PIB has relatively high sensitivity for the detection of amyloid plaques in human brains in vivo (25) and several studies demonstrate significant PIB binding in AD patients as compared to controls (24, 26). About 50 percent of patients with mild cognitive impairment are PIB positive. Significant PIB binding can also be found in about 22 percent of cognitive unimpaired elderly, again supporting the finding that plaques accumulate before cognitive symptoms appear (*9*). Nevertheless, PIB retention during AD progression does not increase to much extend (*27*).

During the recent years, CSF samples of subjects with probable AD were assayed for total or monomeric Aβ40 or Aβ42 concentrations using classical ELISA or ELISA-related methods with additional signal amplification. CSF concentrations of monomeric Aβ42 are reduced by 30 to 50 percent in AD patients compared to age-matched non-demented controls as confirmed in many independent studies, with both sensitivity and specificity exceeding 80 % in most of the studies. Decrease of Aβ42 in the CSF has also been detected during stages of mild cognitive impairment, the earliest clinical manifestation of AD in a subset of individuals and also in individuals with very mild and mild Alzheimer's (*23, 24, 28, 29*). Thus, it was suggested that low levels of CSF Aβ42 might be useful for preclinical diagnosis.

Aβ monomer concentrations in blood were also investigated in several studies. Blood-based biomarkers would be valuable as blood is less complicated to collect than CSF. Unlike changes in the CSF, reports of changes in Aβ levels of plasma in AD patients and non/pre AD are rather inconsistent, which might be due to technical reasons (for reviews see (*28, 30*).

However, the monomeric form of Aβ is not thought to be responsible for neurotoxicity and neurodegeneration. Aβ monomers are a natural metabolic product also abundant in healthy humans and hence a natural component of serum and plasma (*31*). More than Aβ deposits in the brain - the hallmark of AD - Aβ oligomers were identified to be the most toxic species, which arise early in the disease progress. It was shown that the amount of Aβ oligomers in the brain correlates well with cognitive impairment (*18-21*).

PET is currently available in specialized centers only and comparably expensive. It is known to detect amyloid plaques, but not oligomers (*32, 33*). According to Jack and co-workers, the first biomarker change detectable with currently available methods is the decrease of CSF Aβ42, which might reflect the formation of Aβ oligomers and smaller aggregates. This change is followed by amyloid deposition which can be visualized using PIB-PET (*34*).

Therefore, the presence of Aβ oligomers can be expected to be a very early and direct disease biomarker for AD and increasing effort is being made in the development of methods suitable for the detection of Aβ oligomers in body fluids like CSF and plasma.

Here, we review the current status of assay development to reliably and routinely detect Aβ oligomers in body fluids like CSF and blood. Technical progress was severely hampered by the low concentration of Aβ oligomers in body fluids (less than 1 pM (*35*)) and the difficult nature of oligomer versus monomer detection per se. Additionally, we compare the outcomes of the different assay systems and will discuss the drawbacks and opportunities.

Methods for Detection of Aβ Oligomers in Body Fluids

Detection of One Signal for Oligomers

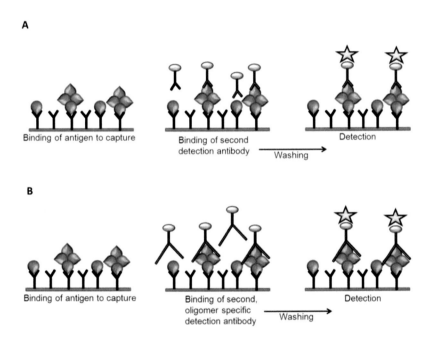

Figure 1. Sandwich ELISA methods for specific Aβ oligomer detection. A: The same antibody is used as a capture and for detection. At least a dimer is required to produce a signal. B: Oligomer specific antibodies in the detection process prevent detection of Aβ monomers.

In recent years, nanotechnology based tools, ELISA-based tools and one mass spectroscopy tool were developed and tested on body fluid samples of AD cases versus non demented controls. All tools described here are based on Aβ caption using specific antibodies. To provide oligomer specificity, either oligomer specific antibodies are employed, or the same general Aβ antibodies were used twice in the system, as capture and for detection. This ensures that only multimers (dimers as smallest detectable unit) of Aβ, but no monomers are detected (see Fig. 1).

All methods described in this part of the chapter are summarized in Table 1. More ELISA methods for Aβ oligomer detection were already described, but to date only applied to brain extract samples (*36-39*). Those are not reviewed here, as the applicability of these assays for body fluids still is to be proven.

Today, three articles are published, which describe the determination of Aβ oligomer concentrations in CSF by "sandwich" methods, with or without additional signal amplification. In 2003, it has been demonstrated that ADDLs ("Aβ derived diffusible ligands", referring to small soluble Aβ oligomers with molecular weights between 17 and 42 kDa (*18*)), were present at significantly elevated levels in brain samples from deceased AD patients (*46*), suggesting that those oligomers might also be found in lower concentrations in CSF. In 2005, two articles about nanoparticle-based assays for the quantitation of ADDLs in CSF were published.

Haes et al. developed and applied a nanoscale optical biosensor method based on localized surface plasmon resonance (LSPR) spectroscopy combined with Aβ oligomer specific antibodies, which was useful to monitor the interaction between ADDLs and ADDL-specific antibodies. In short, ADDL-specific polyclonal antibodies M71 (*47*) were attached to surface-confined silver (Ag) nanoparticles. Subsequently, the nanoparticles were exposed to samples containing ADDLs or control samples. To enhance the LSPR shift response, the samples were incubated a second time with ADDL M71 antibodies (sandwich principle). Transmission UV-vis spectroscopy was used to monitor the optical properties (LSPR) of the Ag nanoparticles. In a very preliminary study, the CSF of one AD patient had a higher concentration of ADDLs than the CSF of one control. These preliminary results were interpreted that LSPR nanosensor technology could be useful as a screening method for human samples and possibly for disease diagnosis (*35*). After that first publication, no subsequent articles referring to the method in combination with ADDL detection were published.

About the same time, Georganopoulou et al. came up with an ultrasensitive barcode assay for the detection of ADDLs in CSF samples. For the assay, oligonucleotide ("barcode")-modified gold nanoparticles as well as magnetic microparticles were functionalized with anti-ADDL antibodies (polyclonal M90 and monoclonal 20C2) and added to the ADDL containing samples.

Table 1. Summary of methods for oligomer detection

Method	Description	Oligomer species detected	Samples	Results	Reference
Nanoscale optical biosensor	Polyclonal anti-oligomer antibody for immobilization and read-out	ADDLs	CSF, Brain extracts, 1 control, 1 AD	Higher ADDL concentration in AD sample	Haes et al., 2005 (35)
Nanoparticle based detection	Polyclonal / monoclonal anti-oligomer antibody for immobilization and read-out	ADDLs	CSF, 15 AD, 15 controls	Higher ADDL concentration in AD samples	Georganopoulou et al., 2005 (40)
ELISA	Monoclonal antibody 13C3 for a protofibrilar form of Aβ42	Protofibrils	Plasma, 1125 elderly without dementia, 104 developed AD after 4.6 years, 402 were tested for protofibrillar Aβ	Decreased protofibrillar Aβ levels with onset of cognitive impairment	Schupf et al., 2008 (41)
ELISA	Same N-terminal antibody used for antigen capture and detection	Oligomers	Plasma and postmortem brain tissue, 26 AD cases, 10 controls	Relative oligomer Aβ levels closely associated to relative Aβ42 levels, decrease of both in AD patients over a 1-to 2-year period	Xia et al., 2009 (42)
ELISA	Same Aβ antibody (BAN 50) used for both antigen capture and detection	HMW oligomers	CSF, 18 AD, 7 MCI, 25 controls	Significantly higher signals in AD or MCI samples, inverse correlation to MMSE scores	Fukumoto et al., 2010 (43)
Method	Description	Oligomer species detected	Samples	Results	Reference
SELDI-TOF incorporating capture antibody	Capture antibody: General Aβ 4G8 or WO2	Dimer	Whole blood, 52 controls, 23 MCI, 43 AD	Significantly higher numer of monomers and dimers in the blood of AD patients, levels correlated with clinical markers	Villemagne et al., 2010 (44)

Definitions of different Aβ species. ADDLs: Aβ derived diffusible ligands small soluble Aβ oligomers with molecular weights between 17 and 42 kDa (18). Protofibrils: ≥ 100 nm curved linear structures with a diameter of ~ 5 nm and a length up to 200 nm which remain soluble upon centrifugation at 16, 000-18,000 x g (45). Aβ oligomers: non fibrillar, soluble low-molecular weight oligomers. HMW oligomers: oligomers of 20-40 kDa (43). Designations describing certain Aβ species are used as by the authors of the reviewed methods. MMSE: Mini-Mental-State-Examination

By means of the antibodies, DNA-ADDL-magnet complexes are formed and could be extracted from the samples using a magnet. Because there are several hundreds of barcodes for each ADDL which was captured, the number of barcodes can be determined after hybridization by scanometric detection methods. Finally, the level of ADDLs in the sample can be calculated. A scheme of bio-barcode assays can be found in Figure 2.

Bio-barcode assays were already proven to be extraordinary sensitive. In a previous report, antigens could be detected with six orders of magnitude greater compared to conventional ELISAs for the same target (48), probably making the assay well suited for applications in AD biomarker development. The detection limit of the semi-quantitative assay was determined to be 100 aM, and the assay was linear up to concentrations of 500 fM. After the assay was established, ADDL concentrations of the CSF samples of 15 AD cases, verified by autopsy, were tested to be consistently higher than the levels of the CSF of non-demented, age matched controls. The ADDL concentration medians were ≈ 200 aM for the controls and 1.7 fM for the AD cases. Only two AD diagnosed individuals showed overlap, what was discussed as possible false positives of previous diagnostic methods. This study was one of the earliest to prove that soluble ADDLs, which were already detected in the brain in earlier studies, can also be found in the CSF, but in very low concentrations. However, similar as described above for the nanoscale optical biosensor, no follow-up articles were published yet.

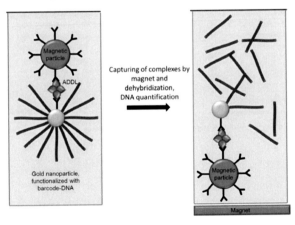

Figure 2. The principle of bio-barcode assays. Antibody conjugated gold nanoparticles with hundreds of DNA barcodes attached, and magnetic beads are functionalized with antibodies that are specific for ADDLs. The DNA-magnet-sandwich complexes are extracted from the sample using a magnet. Subsequently, the total number of DNA barcodes is determined and can be used for the calculation of ADDL levels.

In 2010, Kamali-Moghaddam et al. published an oligomer specific detection assay which was also based on signal amplification. In a sandwich-like assay, binding of protofibrils to the protofibril selective antibody mAb158 was linked to translation of detected signals to amplifiable DNA strands (proximity ligation assay). It allowed detection of 0.1 pg/ml Aβ protofibrils with a high dynamic range, but was so far not used for characterization of Aβ protofibrils in body fluids (49).

Fukumoto et al. developed a novel ELISA specific for high molecular weight (HMW) Aβ oligomers. The same antibody, BAN50 (50), which binds to the N-terminal residues 1 to 16 of Aβ, was used for antigen capture as well as detection. For characterization of the oligomer species detected by the assay, different fractions of synthetic Aβ 42 oligomers were prepared by size exclusion chromatography. The size of the oligomers, which were detected, were determined to be 40 to 200 kDa, mainly fractionating at 45 to 90 kDa, that means mainly 10 to 20 mers. Monomers and lower molecular weight oligomer species were not detected. The detecton limit of the HMW oligomers were 10 pM, expressed as the equivalent concentration of Aβ monomers at the beginning of the preparation. As the HMW oligomers were estimated to be only 1 percent of the whole preparation, the sensitivity of the assay was estimated to be finally 0.1 pM. Why the assay does not detect low molecular weight oligomers like dimers and trimers is not clear yet, but could be due to sterical hindrance.

During application, the authors detected significantly higher amounts of HMW Aβ oligomers in CSF samples from AD and MCI patients as compared to age matched controls. Additionally, the authors could show a negative correlation with MMSE scores in the AD/MCI group. Due to the low concentration of HMW oligomers in the control group (estimated 0.47 pM), the precise HMW oligomers species detected in CSF could not be further characterized (43).

Next to the articles about Aβ oligomer detection in CSF samples, several methods were developed to determine the concentration of Aβ oligomers in plasma or whole blood samples.

In 2008, Schupf et al. investigated how plasma Aβ42, Aβ40 and a protofibrillar subspecies of Aβ42 changed over time and with the onset of dementia or AD. 1125 elderly people without detectable signs of dementia were tested, 104 thereof developed dementia or AD over 4.6 years of follow-up. Conversion to AD was strongly correlated to a decline of Aβ42 levels and of the Aβ42/Aβ40 ratio. In a subset of 402 participants, the levels of Aβ protofibrillar species were determined using a newly developed anti-protofibrillar monoclonal antibody 13C3 in ELISA studies. The authors observed that protofibrillar Aβ could be observed in only 34 % of the participants. The highest levels of protofibrillar Aβ could be detected in individuals with the highest plasma Aβ40 and Aβ42 levels. The decline of protofibrillar, but not soluble Aβ was associated with conversion to mild AD. The authors concluded that decline of Aβ42 species reflects compartmentalization of Aβ in the brain with onset of AD, protofibrillar Aβ being strongly correlated to the onset of cognitive impairment (*41*).

In 2009, Xia et al. published studies about a specific ELISA for detection of Aβ oligomers in plasma and brain tissue of AD patents and controls. To detect Aβ oligomeric species, an ELISA system was applied in which the same antibody (either 82E1 or 3D6) was used as capture and for detection. The assay was established using dimeric, covalently cross-linked, and monomeric Aβ species as negative control and was described to be in a linear fashion and sensitive up to the picomolar range. Disruption of the disulfide bonds of the dimers using β-mercaptoethanol led to markedly reduced signals of the dimers. Monomeric Aβ was not detected.

The oligomer specific assay was used to characterize plasma samples obtained from 36 AD patients and 10 controls, in comparison to conventional Aβ monomer ELISAs. The ages of the AD patients ranged from 50 to 90 years (average age 72 years), those of the controls from 52 to 68 years (average age 62 years). 7 of 10 control subjects had Aβ oligomer levels below the detection limit of the assay, whereas 19 of 36 AD patients had detectable levels of oligomeric Aβ. The authors could not observe an age dependent alteration of Aβ oligomers. Subjects with increased plasma Aβ oligomer concentration ranged from 60 to 90 years. Plasma levels of Aβ42 and oligomeric Aβ species were strongly correlated across the subjects, a similar finding to the one by Schupf et al. A close association between monomeric Aβ42 and oligomeric Aβ42 was suggested. Additionally, a decrease of both levels over a 1- to 2-year period was revealed by the sequential testing of the plasma samples of a subset of AD patients, including a subject with a presenilin mutation and familiar AD. In brain tissue from 9 AD patients, as verified by authopsy, both the Aβ levels of oligomers and monomers were significantly enhanced in comparison to controls. Among all the tested subjects, enhanced levels of oligomeric Aβ were not associated to decreased levels of monomeric Aβ, therefore, the conversion of monomeric Aβ into oligomeric Aβ seems to be not the major contributor to the observed reduction of monomeric Aβ (*42*).

Very recently, Villemagne et al. developed a method for the detection of blood-borne Aβ dimers (*44*). Aβ covalently linked dimers obtained a lot of attraction in the Alzheimer's research field. Aβ dimers were detected in the brains of AD cases, but not in the controls, and were postulated to be the earliest toxic Aβ species (*51, 52*). Whole blood samples were pre-treated with 8 M urea and 0.5 % Triton X-100 and fractionated into plasma and the cellular element fraction (CE). The membrane-rich CE fraction may contain oligomeric Aβ species, as some of the deleterious effects of Aβ could be due to the interaction of oligomeric Aβ species and membranes (*53, 54*). Denaturants and detergents were added to break up potential protein/protein or protein/membrane interactions, which could keep Aβ inaccessible to the capture antibodies used in the process. Aβ in the pre-treated samples was immobilized to the surface of protein chip arrays using the generic Aβ antibodies 4G8 or WO2. Chips were analyzed employing surface enhanced laser desorption ionization-time of flight mass spectrometry (SELDI-TOF). Linear standard curves of concentration versus peak intensity were constructed for synthetic Aβ monomers and dimers to demonstrate that the detected peak was proportional to the sample concentration. The spectra of the plasma fraction did not resolve any peaks which were different between AD and control groups, whereas the spectra of the CE fractions contained a large number of peaks, more than 10 of which were substantially different in the spectra generated from AD samples and controls. The intensities of the peaks generated from Aβ42 monomers were higher as compared to controls by trend, that finding, however did not reach statistical significance. The mass of Aβ dimers was found to be significantly increased in AD compared to control subjects. A strong correlation between the amount of monomeric Aβ and dimers could be detected. The dimer peak was significantly higher in the CE of AD patients when 4G8 was used as capturing antibody (binding epitope amino acid residues 17-24 in comparison to 4-8 for WO2). Elevated Aβ42 and dimer levels in the CE fraction of the blood also correlated with clinical measures of AD, like brain Aβ burden, as measured with PIB, MMSE, memory impairment, executive function and gray matter volume (*44*).

Single Aβ Oligomer Detection

While the methods described above generate one signal summarized for all Aβ oligomers present in the sample volume, this chapter describes methods, in which single aggregates can be detected and, in some of the methods, even characterized in more detail. For single particle detection techniques, methods based on fluorescence correlation spectroscopy (FCS), confocal laser scanning microscopy (LSM) and flow cytometry are applied, all methods principally providing single particle sensitivity. Therefore, in theory, these methods should be even more sensitive than the methods described in the previous chapter.

In 1998, Pitschke et al. published the first method for single Aβ aggregate detection. The method was based on fluorescence correlation spectroscopy (FCS), a method in which particles can be detected in concentrations of less than 100 nM. Fluorescence dye labeled molecules are analyzed in a volume less than a femtoliter, the volume being delimited by confocal illumination with a laser and image formation on a small pinhole in front of extremely sensitive detectors. Labeled Aβ monomers were added to pre-existing multimeric particles in the sample. Based on the principle of seeded polymerization, the labeled monomers should rapidly bind to the pre-existing seeds (for a scheme see Figure 3).

Table 2. Summary of methods for single oligomer detection

Method	Description	Oligomer species detected	Samples	Results	Reference
FCS	Principle of seeded polymerization in combination with FCS	Aβ multimers	CSF, 15 AD, 19 controls	Higher aggregate content in AD-patient derived CSF	Pitschke et al., 1998 (55)
FCS and LSM	Principle of seeded polymerization in combination with FCS + LSM	Aβ binding particles (LAPs)	CSF, 14 AD, 13 other dementia, 6 controls	No correlation found	Henkel et al., 2007 (56)
FRET	Dual colour FRET detection with flow cytometry in solution	Aβ oligomers	CSF, 174 non-demented	Not determined	Navarette-Santos et al., 2007 (57)
Immuno-precipitation	Immunoprecipitation with flow cytometry in solution	Aβ oligomers	Plasma, 17 AD, 16 controls	Higher oligomer concentration in AD samples	Navarette-Santos et al., 2008 (58)
Surface-FIDA	Dual colour single aggregate FCS or LSM detection after immobilization of aggregates	Aβ aggregates	3 AD, 2 controls	Higher aggregate content in AD-patient derived CSF	Funke et al., 2007; Funke et al., 2008; Funke et al., 2010 (59-61)

Definitions of different Aβ multimer species: Aβ oligomers: non fibrillar, soluble low-molecular weight oligomers. Designations describing certain Aβ species are used as by the authors of the reviewed methods. FCS: fluorescence correlation spectroscopy. LSM: laser scanning microscopy. FRET: fluorescence resonance energy transfer.

The fluorescence labeled Aβ was kept soluble using 0.2 % SDS, which was then diluted in the sample to 0.02 %. The final Aβ concentration was less than 100 nM, below the critical solubility limit. The linearity of the assay was demonstrated using synthetically prepared Aβ aggregates and could be verified to range from 20 ng to 1000 ng oligomer per 20 μl sample volume (55).

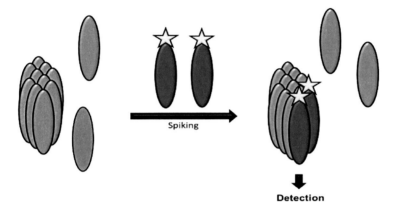

Figure 3. Detection of seeded multimerization. Pre-existing multimeric particles in body fluids are spiked by adding labeled Aβ peptides to the sample. Although the method relies on the conversion (growth) of the original particles in the sample, seeded multimerization is a much faster growth process than spontaneous multimerization. Therefore Aβ oligomers are expected to be preferentially labeled.

CSF samples of 19 non-AD controls produced a fluctuating, but relatively low fluorescence signal in the first 20 min after addition of labeled Aβ, whereas those from 15 AD patients produced high-intensity fluorescence bursts. Each of those peaks was discussed as single oligomeric particle to which fluorescence labeled Aβ was bound. Some rare high intensity bursts in the control group samples were explained by spontaneous aggregation of the fluorescence labeled Aβ or by attachment of fluorescence labeled Aβ to other molecules. The summarized number of fluorescence peaks in the patients was higher than those of the control group, without exception (55).

In 2007, Henkel et al. used a related method to characterize CSF samples of AD patients (n = 14), patients with other dementias (n = 13) and controls (n = 6). Large Aβ-peptide binding particles (LAPs) were detected by spiking samples with fluorescence labeled synthetic Aβ. Thus, the method relies on the conversion (growth) of the original particles in the sample. The sensitivity of detection was improved employing a microtunnel flow-through system to detect the fluorescence of a sample in a home-built FCS system.

A Detection by FRET and flow cytometry   **B** Aggregate detection by Surface-FIDA

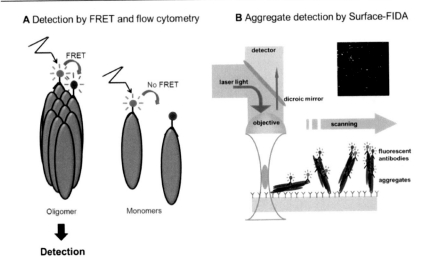

Figure 4. Principles of Aβ oligomer detection by fluorescence resonance energy transfer (FRET) followed by flow cytometry, and Surface-FIDA. A: FRET is a mechanism describing energy transfer between two chromophores. A donor chromophore, initially in its electronic excited state, may transfer energy to an acceptor chromophore in proximity, typically less than 10 nm. Spatial proximity is given between two fluorophors attached to the same Aβ oligomer. The FRET signals are detected by flow cytometry. B: Surface-FIDA is based on a laser focus scanning the surface of a specially prepared glass chip. Either a fluorescence correlation spectroscopy (FCS) device or a laser scanning microscope (LSM) can be used. Aβ aggregates or oligomers are concentrated in a two-dimensional surface by immobilizing them on a glass slide using Aβ capture antibodies. The aggregates are detected after addition of at least two fluorescence-labelled anti-Aβ antibodies. At least two laser beams are focused on the surface of the glass chip and the fluorescence light which is emitted by the fluorescence antibodies is detected in a confocal way, enabling single aggregate detection. The whole surface of the microtiter plate well is scanned in x- and y-directions.

To exclude aggregates solely formed of synthetically prepared, fluorescence labeled Aβ, only bright LAPs (three times the threshold used by Pitschke et al.) were included in the analysis. The binding of fluorescence labeled Aβ to pre-existing particles in the CSF could be verified. Large individual differences could be detected between the patients, but no significant differences in LAP frequency were detected between the groups. The CSF of some patients contained high numbers of LAPs, whereas the samples of others contained virtually none. Confocal laser scanning microscopy (LSM) and a software for integrated morphology analysis was used to image the LAPs and to classify four different subtypes, LAP-1 to LAP-4, based on area, brightness, shape and texture. Autoaggregates composed solely of synthetic Aβ could be clearly defined by heterogenous texture, low brightness and small size. LAP-4 types were particularly interesting, as they could not be detected in any of the AD patients, but they were virtually present in 42.1 % of all non-AD cases. Upon further investigation the authors concluded that LAP-4 particles are aggregates consisting of Aβ and IgGs, assigning a central role to the immune system in Aβ clearance by clustering it in immuncomplexes (55).

In 2007, Navarette Santos et al. described a new approach for single ADDL detection in CSF by a combination of fluorescence resonance energy transfer (FRET) and flow cytometry. FRET means that energy is transferred from an excited donor to an acceptor molecule under favorable spectral and spatial conditions, leading to fluorescence emission of the acceptor molecule. In this special case, Aβ oligomers, termed ADDLs, were labeled by two Aβ antibodies (general Aβ antibodies 4G8 and 6E10), both coupled to fluorescent dyes: Alexa Fluor 488 and Alexa-Fluor 594. In the case that both dyes are in close spatial distance (less than 10 nm), excitation of Alexa 488 and subsequent emission of fluorescent light leads to excitation of the other dye (see Fig. 4A). Subsequently, the FRET events were detected using a FACS cell sorter. When only FRET events are counted, no monomers are detected, and unspecific binding of one of the Aβ antibodies will not lead to a FRET signal. To determine the sensitivity of the assay, ADDLs and fibrils prepared of synthetical Aβ were diluted and analyzed in the procedure. The assay was linear over a range of 10 pM to 2.5 nM, referring to the Aβ monomer concentration. Subsequently, 200 μl human CSF samples of 174 non-demented individuals were analyzed. Evaluation of the data demonstrated a large variation in the concentration of the detected oligomers and a weak correlation between the age of the individuals and the ADDL concentration. The reproducibility of the assay was very high (57). To date, however, no results were published about application of the assay to analyze CSF samples derived from AD patients.

Instead, one year later the authors presented an assay for plasma samples, based on a similar principle of detection. The method combined immunoprecipitation using specific antibodies for different Aβ isoforms with flow cytometry. Aβ in plasma samples in a detergent containing buffer was purified using the general Aβ antibodies 4G8 and 6E10 and goat anti mouse coated beads. The beads were immobilized with a magnetic separator, washed, aliquoted and specifically precipitated with rabbit anti-Aβ40 or rabbit Aβ42 antibodies. The immunoprecipitated complexes were labeled with goat anti rabbit antibody, attached to the fluorescent dye Alexa 488. The detection of different Aβ isoforms was performed using flow cytometry. Plasma samples of

17 AD patients and 16 non-demented controls were subjected to the assay. The results allowed differentiation between the two groups and a specificity and sensitivity of 81.2 and 70.6 % were calculated. This study was the first to demonstrate Aβ oligomer detection in blood, even enabling to estimate the amounts of Aβ oligomer composing isoforms (58).

In 2006 and 2007, Birkmann et al. published a method for the detection of single prion protein (PrP) aggregates prepared from brain samples and in CSF, based on FCS (62, 63). Later, the method was adapted to Aβ aggregates, as described by Funke et al. in 2007 and 2008 (59, 60). The aggregates are immobilized on the surface of a glass chip using an Aβ specific capture, e.g. a general Aβ binding antibody 6E10. The aggregates are then labeled by two different, fluorescence dye coupled antibodies, e.g. 6E10-Alexa 488 and Nab-Alexa 633. Subsequently, the surface of the glass chip is washed and scanned by the laser focus of a FCS system (see Fig. 4B for scheme of assay procedure). As several antibodies bind to one aggregate, aggregates lead to relatively high fluorescence bursts in the FCS confocal detection volume and can thus be easily distinguished from monomers. Additionally, monomer detection can be excluded by use of the same antibody for capturing and detection. As at least two different Aβ antibodies are used in the detection process, the method is highly specific. Only crosscorrelation events are counted as oligomers. The linearity of the assay was evaluated using synthetically prepared aggregated Aβ. The assay was shown to be linear over a wide range of Aβ aggregate amounts to the pg range. As a first trial to use the Surface-FIDA assay for analyzing real CSF samples, 20 µl crude CSF samples of three AD patients and two non-demented control patients were subjected to the assay. The CSF of the AD patients could be clearly distinguished from the control patients. The count of Aβ aggregates was higher in AD patients than in healthy controls (59, 60). Recently, the assay could be optimized with regard to its biochemical steps and adapted to LSM, leading to further improvement of sensitivity. Additionally, now every single aggregate can be characterized with regard to its size and composition (64).

Discussion and Outlook

Very recently, the interest of the Alzheimer's research community to detect Aβ oligomers and aggregates in body fluids grew amazingly. Aβ aggregates, such as soluble Aβ oligomer species, have the potential to be a more suitable biomarker for disease severity and progression than currently measured monomeric CSF Aβ. The development of techniques for the reliable detection and quantitation of aggregated Aβ species, however, is technically challenging due to the heterogenous nature of such aggregates, and their tendency to react further with themselves and with different other proteins. Aβ aggregates can be expected to be abundant in very low concentrations. An additional challenge for the analytical systems is to reliably count only those aggregates or oligomers that consist of Aβ. Monomeric molecules need to be clearly distinguished from oligomers, because Aβ is a normal product of APP metabolism and hence a non-pathologic component of CSF and plasma (65).

Conventional approaches to determine Aβ oligomer levels have been semi-quantitative sodium dodecyl sulfate-polyacrylamid gels and western blotting with subsequent staining of proteins. Those methods, however, are not convenient for diagnostic characterization of minute aggregate concentrations. The development of quantitative techniques for aggregate detection has been promoted by the development of highly sensitive and specific antibodies for Aβ and especially oligomers thereof, and has led to the generation of a couple of methods for aggregate detection.

In the first part of this chapter, several methods for aggregate detection have been described which deliver one signal for all aggregates as an output. Examples are ELISA and "sandwich" based assays with additional signal amplification, or mass spectrometry. In some of those methods, only one form of Aβ conformers is detected as oligomer- or protofibril-specific antibodies are used in those assays. Depending on the probe, such assays will only detect one certain specie of aggregates or will not be able to discriminate between all detected ones. Since the identity of the most relevant Aβ aggregates for AD diagnosis or prognosis is currently an active and controversial research topic, it would require additional evidence to support the use of such assays for diagnostic application. Additionally, care needs to be taken to characterize these antibodies regarding their cross-reactivity with other Aβ aggregate species and monomers.

Especially ELISA assays seem to possess a lot of advantages, as they are easy to perform and technically simple in comparison to other assay forms which were described. Methods like nanoscale optical biosensors and bio-barcode assays, however, promise higher sensitivity, but the reported protocols often contain several critical steps. Those methods may thus have limitations for widespread use as the reported protocols contain e.g. incubation of the sample at 37 °C under shaking, which could lead to massive changes of the oligomerization status of the Aβ pool during the preparation and measurement process, at the end probably limiting the reproducibility of the assay. Another drawback of some of the assays might be the use of polyclonal antibodies, which might lead to poorer reproducibility. Additionally, polyclonal antibodies might not be available in quantities large enough for parallel application of the assay methods in several centers.

In the second part of this chapter, assays are described which allow detection of single aggregates, based on confocal spectroscopy. Some of those assays even permit imaging and further characterization of each single aggregate with regard to aggregate size, form, texture and composition. Characterizations thereof might lead at the end to a better understanding of AD pathology. Some of the assays seem to be very complex and their robustness will have to be proven in future.

As today indicated by five different (preliminary) studies, the count of Aβ aggregates was higher in CSF of AD patients than in healthy controls (*35, 40, 43, 55, 59*). These results further strengthen the theory that Aβ oligomers might be a valuable marker for AD diagnosis and for therapy monitoring as well. In blood, two studies elucidated in this chapter obtained similar results, i.e. increase of Aβ oligomer concentration in samples of AD patients (*44, 58*). However, especially in blood or plasma samples, the results are inconsistent as other studies reported on decreased Aβ oligomer levels with onset of dementia (*41, 42*). These incoherent results can easily be explained by different measurement technologies or by differences in sample preparation. It was already reported that standard operation procedures for sample preparation might lead to more consistent results (*66, 67*). Different steps in blood processing especially influence plasma Aβ detection, as reviewed by Vanderstichele et al. (*68*). Additionally, all results described to date should be considered as preliminary, as they are not statistically significant because of the low numbers of samples which were tested.

In future, a lot of samples will have to be measured with different assay systems to obtain reliable results. Parallel work is needed to elucidate the nature of the Aβ oligomers relevant to the disease as well as to improve the technical robustness of the applied quantification methods. In addition, the question needs to be addressed, whether methods based on antibodies specific for a certain kind of Aβ oligomer or methods that are able to quantify all kinds of Aβ oligomers are suitable to deliver the most valuable biomarker readout. Possibly, a combination of these methods or a completely new so far unknown approach will make it at the end into clinical use.

References

[1] Brookmeyer R, Johnson E, Ziegler-Graham K, Arrighi HM. Forecasting the global burden of Alzheimer's disease. *Alzheimers & Dementia.* 2007 Jul;3(3):186-91.

[2] Folstein MF, Folstein SE, McHugh PR. "Mini-mental state". A practical method for grading the cognitive state of patients for the clinician. *J Psychiatr Res.* 1975 Nov;12(3):189-98.

[3] Mohs RC, Cohen L. Alzheimer's Disease Assessment Scale (ADAS). *Psychopharmacol Bull.* 1988;24(4):627-8.

[4] Knopman DS, DeKosky ST, Cummings JL, Chui H, Corey-Bloom J, Relkin N, et al. Practice parameter: diagnosis of dementia (an evidence-based review). Report of the Quality Standards Subcommittee of the American Academy of Neurology. *Neurology.* 2001 May 8;56(9):1143-53.

[5] Visser PJ, Scheltens P, Verhey FR. Do MCI criteria in drug trials accurately identify subjects with predementia Alzheimer's disease? *J Neurol Neurosurg Psychiatry.* 2005 Oct;76(10):1348-54.

[6] Ganguli M, Rodriguez E, Mulsant B, Richards S, Pandav R, Bilt JV, et al. Detection and management of cognitive impairment in primary care: The Steel Valley Seniors Survey. *J Am Geriatr Soc.* 2004 Oct;52(10):1668-75.

[7] Braak H, Braak E. Frequency of stages of Alzheimer-related lesions in different age categories. *Neurobiol Aging.* 1997 Jul-Aug;18(4):351-7.

[8] Price JL, McKeel DW, Jr., Buckles VD, Roe CM, Xiong C, Grundman M, et al. Neuropathology of nondemented aging: presumptive evidence for preclinical Alzheimer disease. *Neurobiol Aging.* 2009 Jul;30(7):1026-36.

[9] Mintun MA, Larossa GN, Sheline YI, Dence CS, Lee SY, Mach RH, et al. [11C]PIB in a nondemented population: potential antecedent marker of Alzheimer disease. *Neurology.* 2006 Aug 8;67(3):446-52.

[10] Jakob-Roetne R, Jacobsen H. Alzheimer's disease: from pathology to therapeutic approaches. *Angew Chem Int Ed Engl.* 2009;48(17):3030-59.

[11] Nerelius C, Johansson J, Sandegren A. Amyloid beta-peptide aggregation. What does it result in and how can it be prevented? *Front Biosci.* 2009;14:1716-29.

[12] Finder VH, Glockshuber R. Amyloid-beta aggregation. *Neurodegener Dis.* 2007;4(1):13-27.

[13] Kang J, Lemaire HG, Unterbeck A, Salbaum JM, Masters CL, Grzeschik KH, et al. The precursor of Alzheimer's disease amyloid A4 protein resembles a cell-surface receptor. *Nature.* 1987 Feb 19-25;325(6106):733-6.

[14] Weidemann A, Konig G, Bunke D, Fischer P, Salbaum JM, Masters CL, et al. Identification, biogenesis, and localization of precursors of Alzheimer's disease A4 amyloid protein. *Cell.* 1989 Apr 7;57(1):115-26.

[15] Haass C, Selkoe DJ. Cellular processing of beta-amyloid precursor protein and the genesis of amyloid beta-peptide. *Cell.* 1993 Dec 17;75(6):1039-42.

[16] Hardy JA, Higgins GA. Alzheimer's disease: the amyloid cascade hypothesis. *Science.* 1992 Apr 10;256(5054):184-5.

[17] Selkoe DJ. The molecular pathology of Alzheimer's disease. *Neuron.* 1991 Apr;6(4):487-98.

[18] Lambert MP, Barlow AK, Chromy BA, Edwards C, Freed R, Liosatos M, et al. Diffusible, nonfibrillar ligands derived from Abeta1-42 are potent central nervous system neurotoxins. *Proc Natl Acad Sci U S A.* 1998 May 26;95(11):6448-53.

[19] Haass C, Selkoe DJ. Soluble protein oligomers in neurodegeneration: lessons from the Alzheimer's amyloid beta-peptide. *Nat Rev Mol Cell Biol.* 2007 Feb;8(2):101-12.

[20] Shankar GM, Bloodgood BL, Townsend M, Walsh DM, Selkoe DJ, Sabatini BL. Natural oligomers of the Alzheimer amyloid-beta protein induce reversible synapse loss by modulating an NMDA-type glutamate receptor-dependent signaling pathway. *J Neurosci.* 2007 Mar 14;27(11):2866-75.

[21] Walsh DM, Selkoe DJ. A beta oligomers - a decade of discovery. *J Neurochem.* 2007 Jun;101(5):1172-84.

[22] Nordberg A, Rinne JO, Kadir A, Langstrom B. The use of PET in Alzheimer disease. *Nat Rev Neurol.* Feb;6(2):78-87.

[23] Blennow K, Zetterberg H. Is it time for biomarker-based diagnostic criteria for prodromal Alzheimer's disease? *Alzheimers Res Ther.*2(2):8.

[24] Fagan AM, Holtzman DM. Cerebrospinal fluid biomarkers of Alzheimer's disease. *Biomark Med.* Feb;4(1):51-63.

[25] Edison P, Archer HA, Hinz R, Hammers A, Pavese N, Tai YF, et al. Amyloid, hypometabolism, and cognition in Alzheimer disease: an [11C]PIB and [18F]FDG PET study. *Neurology.* 2007 Feb 13;68(7):501-8.

[26] Berti V, Osorio RS, Mosconi L, Li Y, De Santi S, de Leon MJ. Early detection of Alzheimer's disease with PET imaging. *Neurodegener Dis*.7(1-3):131-5.

[27] Engler H, Forsberg A, Almkvist O, Blomquist G, Larsson E, Savitcheva I, et al. Two-year follow-up of amyloid deposition in patients with Alzheimer's disease. *Brain*. 2006 Nov;129(Pt 11):2856-66.

[28] Blennow K, Hampel H, Weiner M, Zetterberg H. Cerebrospinal fluid and plasma biomarkers in Alzheimer disease. *Nat Rev Neurol*. Mar;6(3):131-44.

[29] Hansson O, Zetterberg H, Buchhave P, Londos E, Blennow K, Minthon L. Association between CSF biomarkers and incipient Alzheimer's disease in patients with mild cognitive impairment: a follow-up study. *Lancet Neurol*. 2006 Mar;5(3):228-34.

[30] Thambisetty M, Lovestone S. Blood-based biomarkers of Alzheimer's disease: challenging but feasible. *Biomark Med*. Feb;4(1):65-79.

[31] Lesne S, Koh MT, Kotilinek L, Kayed R, Glabe CG, Yang A, et al. A specific amyloid-beta protein assembly in the brain impairs memory. *Nature*. 2006 Mar 16;440(7082):352-7.

[32] Lockhart A, Lamb JR, Osredkar T, Sue LI, Joyce JN, Ye L, et al. PIB is a non-specific imaging marker of amyloid-beta (Abeta) peptide-related cerebral amyloidosis. *Brain*. 2007 Oct;130(Pt 10):2607-15.

[33] Maeda J, Ji B, Irie T, Tomiyama T, Maruyama M, Okauchi T, et al. Longitudinal, quantitative assessment of amyloid, neuroinflammation, and anti-amyloid treatment in a living mouse model of Alzheimer's disease enabled by positron emission tomography. *J Neurosci*. 2007 Oct 10;27(41):10957-68.

[34] Jack CR, Jr., Knopman DS, Jagust WJ, Shaw LM, Aisen PS, Weiner MW, et al. Hypothetical model of dynamic biomarkers of the Alzheimer's pathological cascade. *Lancet Neurol*. Jan;9(1):119-28.

[35] Haes AJ, Chang L, Klein WL, Van Duyne RP. Detection of a biomarker for Alzheimer's disease from synthetic and clinical samples using a nanoscale optical biosensor. *J Am Chem Soc*. 2005 Feb 23;127(7):2264-71.

[36] Englund H, Sehlin D, Johansson AS, Nilsson LN, Gellerfors P, Paulie S, et al. Sensitive ELISA detection of amyloid-beta protofibrils in biological samples. *J Neurochem*. 2007 Oct;103(1):334-45.

[37] Barghorn S, Nimmrich V, Striebinger A, Krantz C, Keller P, Janson B, et al. Globular amyloid beta-peptide oligomer - a homogenous and stable

neuropathological protein in Alzheimer's disease. *J Neurochem.* 2005 Nov;95(3):834-47.

[38]   Lee EB, Leng LZ, Zhang B, Kwong L, Trojanowski JQ, Abel T, et al. Targeting amyloid-beta peptide (Abeta) oligomers by passive immunization with a conformation-selective monoclonal antibody improves learning and memory in Abeta precursor protein (APP) transgenic mice. *J Biol Chem.* 2006 Feb 17;281(7):4292-9.

[39]   van Helmond Z, Heesom K, Love S. Characterisation of two antibodies to oligomeric Abeta and their use in ELISAs on human brain tissue homogenates. *J Neurosci Methods.* 2009 Jan 30;176(2):206-12.

[40]   Georganopoulou DG, Chang L, Nam JM, Thaxton CS, Mufson EJ, Klein WL, et al. Nanoparticle-based detection in cerebral spinal fluid of a soluble pathogenic biomarker for Alzheimer's disease. *Proc Natl Acad Sci U S A.* 2005 Feb 15;102(7):2273-6.

[41]   Schupf N, Tang MX, Fukuyama H, Manly J, Andrews H, Mehta P, et al. Peripheral Abeta subspecies as risk biomarkers of Alzheimer's disease. *Proc Natl Acad Sci U S A.* 2008 Sep 16;105(37):14052-7.

[42]   Xia W, Yang T, Shankar G, Smith IM, Shen Y, Walsh DM, et al. A specific enzyme-linked immunosorbent assay for measuring beta-amyloid protein oligomers in human plasma and brain tissue of patients with Alzheimer disease. *Arch Neurol.* 2009 Feb;66(2):190-9.

[43]   Fukumoto H, Tokuda T, Kasai T, Ishigami N, Hidaka H, Kondo M, et al. High-molecular-weight {beta}-amyloid oligomers are elevated in cerebrospinal fluid of Alzheimer patients. *FASEB J.* Mar 25.

[44]   Villemagne VL, Perez KA, Pike KE, Kok WM, Rowe CC, White AR, et al. Blood-borne amyloid-beta dimer correlates with clinical markers of Alzheimer's disease. *J Neurosci.* May 5;30(18):6315-22.

[45]   Walsh DM, Klyubin I, Fadeeva JV, Cullen WK, Anwyl R, Wolfe MS, et al. Naturally secreted oligomers of amyloid beta protein potently inhibit hippocampal long-term potentiation in vivo. *Nature.* 2002 Apr 4;416(6880):535-9.

[46]   Gong Y, Chang L, Viola KL, Lacor PN, Lambert MP, Finch CE, et al. Alzheimer's disease-affected brain: presence of oligomeric A beta ligands (ADDLs) suggests a molecular basis for reversible memory loss. *Proc Natl Acad Sci U S A.* 2003 Sep 2;100(18):10417-22.

[47]   Lambert MP, Viola KL, Chromy BA, Chang L, Morgan TE, Yu J, et al. Vaccination with soluble Abeta oligomers generates toxicity-neutralizing antibodies. *J Neurochem.* 2001 Nov;79(3):595-605.

[48] Nam JM, Thaxton CS, Mirkin CA. Nanoparticle-based bio-bar codes for the ultrasensitive detection of proteins. *Science.* 2003 Sep 26;301(5641):1884-6.

[49] Kamali-Moghaddam M, Ekholm Pettersson F, Wu D, Englund H, Darmanis S, Lord A, et al. Sensitive detection of Abeta protofibrils by proximity ligation - relevance for Alzheimer's disease. *BMC Neurosci.* Oct 5;11(1):124.

[50] Suzuki N, Cheung TT, Cai XD, Odaka A, Otvos L, Jr., Eckman C, et al. An increased percentage of long amyloid beta protein secreted by familial amyloid beta protein precursor (beta APP717) mutants. *Science.* 1994 May 27;264(5163):1336-40.

[51] Mc Donald JM, Savva GM, Brayne C, Welzel AT, Forster G, Shankar GM, et al. The presence of sodium dodecyl sulphate-stable Abeta dimers is strongly associated with Alzheimer-type dementia. *Brain.* May;133(Pt 5):1328-41.

[52] Shankar GM, Li S, Mehta TH, Garcia-Munoz A, Shepardson NE, Smith I, et al. Amyloid-beta protein dimers isolated directly from Alzheimer's brains impair synaptic plasticity and memory. *Nat Med.* 2008 Aug;14(8):837-42.

[53] Glabe CG, Kayed R. Common structure and toxic function of amyloid oligomers implies a common mechanism of pathogenesis. *Neurology.* 2006 Jan 24;66(2 Suppl 1):S74-8.

[54] Hung LW, Ciccotosto GD, Giannakis E, Tew DJ, Perez K, Masters CL, et al. Amyloid-beta peptide (Abeta) neurotoxicity is modulated by the rate of peptide aggregation: Abeta dimers and trimers correlate with neurotoxicity. *J Neurosci.* 2008 Nov 12;28(46):11950-8.

[55] Pitschke M, Prior R, Haupt M, Riesner D. Detection of single amyloid beta-protein aggregates in the cerebrospinal fluid of Alzheimer's patients by fluorescence correlation spectroscopy. *Nat Med.* 1998 Jul;4(7):832-4.

[56] Henkel AW, Dittrich PS, Groemer TW, Lemke EA, Klingauf J, Klafki HW, et al. Immune complexes of auto-antibodies against A beta 1-42 peptides patrol cerebrospinal fluid of non-Alzheimer's patients. *Mol Psychiatry.* 2007 Jun;12(6):601-10.

[57] Santos AN, Torkler S, Nowak D, Schlittig C, Goerdes M, Lauber T, et al. Detection of amyloid-beta oligomers in human cerebrospinal fluid by flow cytometry and fluorescence resonance energy transfer. *J Alzheimers Dis.* 2007 Mar;11(1):117-25.

[58] Santos AN, Simm A, Holthoff V, Boehm G. A method for the detection of amyloid-beta1-40, amyloid-beta1-42 and amyloid-beta oligomers in

blood using magnetic beads in combination with Flow cytometry and its application in the diagnostics of Alzheimer's disease. *J Alzheimers Dis.* 2008 Jun;14(2):127-31.

[59] Funke SA, Birkmann E, Henke F, Gortz P, Lange-Asschenfeldt C, Riesner D, et al. Single particle detection of Abeta aggregates associated with Alzheimer's disease. *Biochem Biophys Res Commun.* 2007 Dec 28;364(4):902-7.

[60] Funke SA, Birkmann E, Henke F, Gortz P, Lange-Asschenfeldt C, Riesner D, et al. An ultrasensitive assay for diagnosis of Alzheimer's disease. *Rejuvenation Res.* 2008 Apr;11(2):315-8.

[61] Funke SA, Wang L, Birkmann E, Willbold D. Single-Particle Detection System for Abeta Aggregates: Adaptation of Surface-Fluorescence Intensity Distribution Analysis to Laser Scanning Microscopy. *Rejuvenation Res.* 2010 Apr-Jun;13(2-3):206-9.

[62] Birkmann E, Henke F, Weinmann N, Dumpitak C, Groschup M, Funke A, et al. Counting of single prion particles bound to a capture-antibody surface (surface-FIDA). *Vet Microbiol.* 2007 Aug 31;123(4):294-304.

[63] Birkmann E, Schafer O, Weinmann N, Dumpitak C, Beekes M, Jackman R, et al. Detection of prion particles in samples of BSE and scrapie by fluorescence correlation spectroscopy without proteinase K digestion. *Biol Chem.* 2006 Jan;387(1):95-102.

[64] Funke SA, Birkmann E, Willbold D. Detection of Amyloid-beta aggregates in body fluids: a suitable method for early diagnosis of Alzheimer's disease? *Curr Alzheimer Res.* 2010 Jun;6(3):285-9.

[65] Haass C, Schlossmacher MG, Hung AY, Vigo-Pelfrey C, Mellon A, Ostaszewski BL, et al. Amyloid beta-peptide is produced by cultured cells during normal metabolism. *Nature.* 1992 Sep 24;359(6393):322-5.

[66] Lewczuk P, Beck G, Ganslandt O, Esselmann H, Deisenhammer F, Regeniter A, et al. International quality control survey of neurochemical dementia diagnostics. *Neurosci Lett.* 2006 Nov 27;409(1):1-4.

[67] Bjerke M, Portelius E, Minthon L, Wallin A, Anckarsater H, Anckarsater R, et al. Confounding factors influencing amyloid Beta concentration in cerebrospinal fluid. *Int J Alzheimers Dis.*2010.

[68] Vanderstichele H, Van Kerschaver E, Hesse C, Davidsson P, Buyse MA, Andreasen N, et al. Standardization of measurement of beta-amyloid(1-42) in cerebrospinal fluid and plasma. *Amyloid.* 2000 Dec;7(4):245-58.

In: Alzheimer's Diagnosis   ISBN: 978-1-61209-846-3
Editor: Charles E. Ronson, pp. 25-41   ©2011 Nova Science Publishers, Inc.

Chapter II

Visual Impairment in Alzheimer Disease: Clinical, Pathophysiological and Instrumental Aspects

Ferdinando Sartucci[*,1,2,3], *Tommaso Bocci*[1,4],
Elisa Giorli[1,4], *Vittorio Porciatti*[5], *Nicola Origlia*[2]
and Luciano Domenici[2,6]

[1]Neuroscience Department, Unit of Neurology,
Pisa University Medical School, Pisa;
[2] CNR Neuroscience Institute, Pisa;
[3]S.D. Outpatient Neurological Activity, AOUP, Pisa, Italy;
[4]Department of Neuroscience, Neurology and Clinical Neurophysiology
Section, Siena University Medical School,
Siena, Italy;
[5] Bascom Palmer Eye Institute, Miami, FL, USA;
[6]Department of Biomedical Sciences and Technologies,
L'Aquila University, L'Aquila, Italy

[*] Associate Professor of Neurology, Pisa University Medical School; Neuroscience Department,
Unit of Neurology, Via Roma, n. 67; I 56126 - Pisa (Italy), Phones: +39.050.996760
(direct), 996767 (secretary office); Fax: +39.050. 996767, E-Mail: f.sartucci@neuro.med.
unipi.it, Secretary: m.santin@ao-pisa.toscana.it, http://www.unipi.it

Introduction

Alzheimer's Disease (AD) is the most common cause of dementia in the older adults world-wide. About 4.5 million individuals in USA currently are estimated to be affected and by mid-century the prevalence will be 11.3-16 million cases (Cronin-Golomb and Hof, 2004). AD is viewed as a disorder primarily of memory, that represents usually the initial sign; moreover, this disease is characterized by impairment in several additional domains, including visual function. However, the NINCDS-ADRDA clinical diagnostic criteria (Tierney et al., 1988) make no mention of sensory changes. Several main fields of researches on vision in AD currently are undertaken, from structure to function and behavior at this time, and current directions in AD vision studies are extensively reported in many papers, including some exhaustive books (Cronin-Golomb and Hof, 2004). In summary, this chapter spans the visual impairment in AD patients, from structure to function, either at retinal or cortical levels in an attempt to highlight visual sub-system changes, particularly the magnocellular, in AD compared to normal aging and other age-related degenerative disorders.

Clinical Aspects

Alzheimer's Disease impairs visual function at an early-intermediate state of degeneration and functional losses correlate with severity of cognitive progressive impairment. Different visual deficits have been reported in AD patients, such as alteration of contrast sensitivity (Cronin-Golomb et al., 1991), motion perception (Gilmore GC, 1994; Duffy et al., 2000), performance on masling tests (Cronin-Golomb et al., 1991), colour discrimination of blue, short-wavelength hues (Cronin-Golomb et al., 1991), visual attention and visual behavior, face discrimination, imagery (Valenti, 2004). In the absence of an accurate biomarker, the diagnosis relies on cognitive profile supported by neuroimaging (Scheltens and Kittner, 2000).

Neuropathological Changes in Alzheimer's Disease: The Visual Variant

In addition to typical form of AD, a growing number of cases of focal cortical presentations has recently been described: in particular, the posterior cortical atrophy (PCA) is commonly accompanied by visuospatial impairment, which recalls the clinical characteristics of both Balint's and Gerstmann's Syndromes; visual agnosia, dressing apraxia, environmental disorientation. PCA presents as biparietal syndrome and tends to remain confined to posterior areas for a very long time before spreading away (Alladi et al., 2007). Patients with PCA are older than those with typical AD and have less memory loss or reduced verbal fluency. Unfortunately, differential diagnosis remains anamnestic, even if modern functional imaging, such as amyloid binding ligand PIB or positron emission tomography with carbon 11 (Ng et al., 2007), could be helpful in the near future to discriminate these pathologies *in vivo*. Moreover, the distribution of senile plaques (SP) and neurofibrillary tangles (NFT) is quite different between typical AD and visuospatial variant. Areas 17, 18 and 19 contain a much higher density of NFT in PCA; in patients with visual agnosia also the regions of inferior temporal cortex and occipitotemporal junction (areas 37, 20 and 21; Von Gunten et al., 2004) show increased deposition of NFT and SP compared to typical AD. These data are consistent with the view that PCA affects the feed-forward projections to high-level regions and to associative visual areas, but the etiopathological bases remain elusive so far.

New Neuropathological Vistas on Alzheimer's Disease: Focus on the Visual System

Extensive deposition of amyloid-β (Aβ) leading to the formation of plaques is considered one of the key pathological features of AD (Gandy, 2005). Aβ derives from the cleavage of amyloid-β protein precursor and exists in a variety of forms including monomers, oligomers, protofibrils, and fibrils (Stromer and Serpell, 2005). Recent observations in both AD patients and AD-type mouse models showed that impairment of memory and synaptic deficit occur prior to extensive extracellular deposition of Aβ in the brain (Hsiao et al., 1996; Hsia et al., 1999; Redwine et al., 2003; Arancio et al., 2004; Jacobsen et al., 2006). Thus, oligomeric Aβ plays an important role in neuronal and synaptic dysfunction during an early phase of AD progression Aβ aggregation and deposition under the form of senile plaques (Selkoe, 2002). Interestingly, in a recent paper by Origlia et al. (Origlia et al., 2009), these authors demonstrated that low concentrations of oligomeric Aβ are capable of disrupting synaptic plasticity in different circuits of the mouse visual cortex. As an intriguing finding long-term synaptic plasticity (LTP) in supragranular horizontal pathways (layer II/III) is altered by lower concentration of Aβ respect to other intracortical pathways (WM-layer II/III vertical pathway). Moreover, different intra-cortical connections that convey specific and distinct aspects of sensory related information necessary for cognitive functions are differently affected by increasing amount of Aβ; for instance, high sensitive horizontal pathway in layer II/III is more closely involved in elaboration and retrieval of previously stored sensory input (Hasselmo and Giocomo, 2006).

The reported results together with previous studies (Hyman et al., 1984; Gomez-Isla et al., 1996) showing the presence of laminar differences within single brain areas in AD progress, raises the important question of whether the pattern of AD reflects the sensitivity of different neurons and/or synaptic connections to pathogens including Aβ.

Alterations in amyloid precursor protein (APP) processing and Aβ accumulation may therefore contribute to retinal damage as well as to cortical alterations as above reported. Several reports outlined the role of oligomeric Aβ in retinal pigmented epithelium (RPE) alterations and dysfunctions, ganglion cells dysfunction, inflammatory and oxidative process till cell death (Bruban et al., 2009; Dutescu et al., 2009); indeed, APP and its products including Aβ were detected in retinal as well as in cerebral extracts from two murine models of AD.

Altogether the reported results permit to advance the hypothesis that visual system, from retina to cortical areas, might be affected during an early-intermediate stage of AD characterized by large absence of SP, NFT and cell death; following this idea an increasing amount of oligomeric beta accumulation induces synaptic toxicity and dysfunction in several cells from retina to cortex. Whether Aβ-dependent visual impairment in AD is due to retinal pathology or due to post-retinal pathology remains unclear.

The Segregation of P- and M-Stream in Humans

The post-receptorial visual pathways of primates contain two major parallel streams specific for colour contrast/form discrimination and luminance contrast/movement discrimination (De Monasterio and Gouras, 1975; Dreher et al., 1976; Shapley, 1990; Van Essen and Gallant, 1994). The colour-opponent system originates from small, tonic ganglion cells relaying to parvocellular laminae of the lateral geniculate nucleus and then projecting to layer 4C-β of the striate cortex. More deeply, recent data showed that two colour-opponent pathways, red-green (RG) and blue-yellow (B-Y), form the so-called parvo- (P) and konio-cellular (K) streams, respectively (Merigan and Maunsell, 1993; Dacey and Lee, 1994; Porciatti and Sartucci, 1999). The second major subsystem, i.e. the achromatic stream, originates from large, phasic ganglion cells projecting to the magnocellular (M) layers of the lateral geniculate nucleus and then to laminae 4C-β of the striate visual cortex (Lennie et al., 1990; Engel et al., 1997). It is worth to note that parvocellular cells may also respond well to achromatic contrast stimuli of relatively high-spatial frequency. However, within the range of spatial frequencies to which both streams respond, M cells are relatively more sensitive to achromatic contrast and this characteristic is more prominent at higher temporal frequencies. To date, it is common knowledge that a specific decline in high-spatial contrast and low-temporal frequency sensitivity suggests a selective deficit in P-stream (Di Russo and Spinelli, 1999), whereas the loss of motion perception and the impairment in analyzing low-spatial frequency and contrast luminance are more likely to be related with severe dysfunction affecting M-pathway. The small receptive fields of the parvo channels in the center of vision yield a strong local motion signal, whereas the magno- ones with their fast transmission time and large receptive fields ensure the integration of global motion signals over a larger area.

From Histopathology to Psychophysiology: New Insights into the Involvement of Magnocellular Stream in Alzheimer's Disease

Histopathological studies demonstrated that hippocampus and the parahippocampal regions are the earliest affected regions in AD, suggesting a hierarchical order of involvement: from limbic to associative cortical areas, from associative to primary sensory cortical areas including the visual cortex (Moore,1997). Following this scheme, the involvement of visual system characterizes a late phase of AD, as well as the non pathological aging (Fiorentini et al., 1996). However, recent studies have highlighted an apparent dichotomy between the progress of histopathological findings in different brain areas and the occurrence of visual dysfunctions in AD patients. In particular, clinical studies support a link between cognitive performance and visual dysfunction even at an early stage of AD when SP and NFT are largely absent. Impairment of higher order visual processing, such as the loss of color discrimination, stereoacuity, contrast sensitivity, and backward masking, have been frequently described in AD patients (Mendez et al., 1990; Cronin-Golomb et al., 1991; Rizzo et al., 2000).

Blanks and colleagues first tried to examine the degeneration of the retinal ganglion cells, finding that cells with largest diameters, by which magnocellular stream is made up, are selectively affected in AD patients (Blanks et al., 1989). Another indirect, but highly convincing data in support of a specific visual impairment come from the study of Dentchev et al. (Dentchev et al., 2003) who emphasized the presence of Aβ proteins in the retina of AD patients compared to nine individuals with age-related macular degeneration and nine age and sex-matched controls.

Hof and Morrison (1990) hypothesized that, even if there is less NFT deposition in the occipital areas than in the prefrontal and temporal cortices, AD patients often exhibit a significant neuronal loss within specific cortical layers, i.e. IV-C and IV-B, where magnocellular stream terminates (Hof and Morrison, 1990); this observation agrees with both a motion perception impairment and an extensive M-pathway dysfunction in AD, possibly caused by oligomeric Aβ accumulation in different cortical layers (Origlia et al., 2009).

Our Experience

Although recent studies suggest that segregation between main visual streams is not complete, the present chapter addresses the hypothesis that AD involves a deficit in the magnocellular pathway of the visual system using ERGs and VEPs to chromatic (Ch, P and K streams) and luminance (Lum, M stream) stimuli. Besides that, electrophysiological analysis of these three different streams might be relatively simple also considering that sensory inputs are conveyed to the LGN, and then to V1 cortical area, in a one-to-one ordered fashion. Previous reports showed that luminance and chromatic contrast sensitivity develop independently at different rates, probably reflecting a different development of postreceptoral neural mechanisms (Brodie et al., 1992; Fiorentini et al., 1996).

We raise the hypothesis that AD involves a deficit in the M-pathway resulting in subtle dysfunction at the level of the retina, post-retinal pathways and/or visual cortex. To this aim we recorded electroretinograms and visual potentials evoked by chromatic and luminance visual stimuli (ChPERGs and

ChVEPs, LumERGs and LumVEPs) in a selected sample of AD patients and compared results with a control group of age and sex matched healthy subjects. AD patients met the diagnostic criteria of probable AD according to the Diagnostic and Statistical Manual of Mental Disorders, fourth edition (DSM-4), the ICD-10 Classification of Mental and Behavioral Disorders (ICD-10) and the criteria of the National Institute of Neurologic and Communicative Disorders and Stroke and the Alzheimer's Disease and Related Disorders Association (NINCDS-ADRDA; McKhann et al., 1984). Severity of dementia was assessed using MMSE (Crum et al., 1993), even if patients have been examined by means of a extensive standardized diagnostic protocol (Tognoni et al., 2005); at the time of diagnosis, all the patients presented a MMSE score below 23/30. Diagnosis of AD was supported by a exhaustive diagnostic work-up including morphological and functional neuroimaging. In particular each patient underwent a brain MRI scan and a FDG-PET semi quantitative study, electroencephalogram and auditory P300 Event Related Potentials (ERPs). Other possible causes of dementia were excluded. The disease onset was homogeneous among patients and disease duration from onset varied from 12 to 16 months; no one case showed a cerebrovascular load more than two minor lacunar microlesions, as proved by neuroimaging. Moreover, we considered as normal small areas of long T2 MRI-imaging around the frontal horns, reflecting either mild and age-related white matter changes or minor ischemic events (Erkinjuntti et al., 1987)

Visual Stimuli

Visual stimuli were equiluminant horizontal sinusoidal gratings, modulated either in luminance (yellow-black, Y-Bk) and chromaticity (red-green, R-G and blue-yellow, B-Y). R-G chromatic gratings were obtained by superimposing (out of phase by 180∘) red-black to green-black luminance gratings, and blue-yellow chromatic grating were obtained by superimposing (also out of phase by 180∘) blue-black to yellow-black luminance gratings. Red-black, green-black, blue-black, and yellow-black luminance gratings had the same Michelson contrast (K) levels (90%), which was used to define the contrast of the chromatic grating. Gratings were generated by a VSG/2 graphic card (Cambridge Research©, UK), displayed full-field on a colour monitor (Samsung Sync Master 1100DF®, 21 inches) at a frame rate of 120 Hz and 14 bits per colour per pixel, suitably linearized by gamma correction (Porciatti and Sartucci, 1996, 1999). The equiluminant point was detected for each subject by assessing contrast sensitivity with the method of ascending limits for a 1 c/deg red-green or black-yellow grating (Fiorentini et al.,, 1996), counterphased at 15 Hz. The point of minimum sensitivity was taken as the equiluminant value for the subject. The relative luminance (r) is easily defined by the formula (Mullen et al., 1985):

$$r = Lum_{red} / Lum_{red} + Lum_{green}$$

where values of r=0, r = 0.5 (equiluminant point, at maximum chromatic contrast) and r = 1.0 respectively define G-Bk, R-G and R-Bk patterns. Red-green gratings were sinusoidally reversed at 16 Hz and the r-ratio was varied to null or minimize the perception of flicker. The extreme values (i.e. r = 0 and r = 1) characterize gratings with pure luminance contrast and poor chromatic one. This implies that, at low-spatial frequencies below 5 cycles/deg, contrast sensitivity is greater to the chromatic gratings, consisting of two monochromatic gratings added in anti-phase, than to monochromatic grating alone. Above 5 cycles/deg, contrast sensitivity is greater to monochromatic than to chromatic gratings. Contrast sensitivity reflects the minimum amount of contrast that an observer needs to resolve a stimulus of a given size.

Results

Transient exemplificative single waveforms and grand average of PERGs and VEPs, obtained either in controls and AD patients, are summarized in Fig. 1 and 2. Our data show evident abnormalities both in latency and amplitude only of Lum PERGs and VEPs in AD patients (filled arrows) compared with controls, while no significant differences were found in chromatic responses between the two groups. VEPs and retino-cortical time (RCT) analysis did not revealed a retinocalcarine pathway involvement associated with AD, suggesting the existence of a specific magnocellular or M-pathway deficit (Sartucci et al., 2010). In AD patients (bottom line of figures), transient PERGs obtained by Y-Bk pattern, had P1 and N1 peak latency with an average of 61.0 ± 5.2 and 96.1 ± 5.8 ms (in controls $38,1\pm2.4$ and 73.4 ± 8.6 respectively; $p \leq 0.01$); a mean amplitude of 0.2 ± 0.3 and $0.36\pm0.59\mu V$ (in controls 0.3 ± 0.2 and 1.5 ± 0.9; $p \leq 0.05$). The VEPs N-wave showed a mean latency of 188.8 ± 8.6ms and a mean amplitude of $3.03\pm0.48\mu V$ (in controls 166.6 ± 6.8 and 3.6 ± 1.2; $p \leq 0.05$).

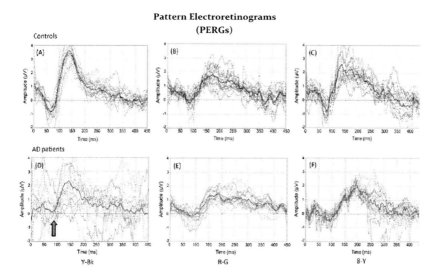

Figure 1. Transient PERGs in response to either Y-Bk luminance grating (A and D), equiluminant chromatic R-G (B and E) and B-Y (C and F) in controls (top traces) and AD patients (bottom traces). For each inset, individual waveform are represented by dotted line, the grand mean by bold line (From Sartucci et al. 2010, with permission).

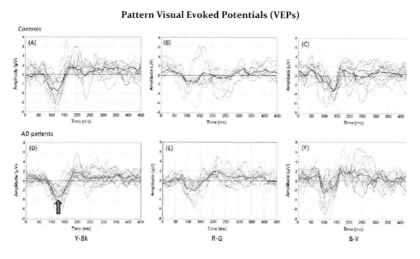

Figure 2. Transient VEPs in response to either Y-Bk luminance grating (A and D), R-G (B and E) and B-Y (C and F) in controls (top traces) and AD patients (bottom traces). As in previous figure, for each inset, individual waveform are represented by dotted line, the grand mean by bold line. Note the latency delay for Y-Bk and B-Y stimuli, whereas R-G are relatively spared (From Sartucci et al. 2010, with permission).

Against a High-Order Visual Impairment as a Primary Marker of Alzheimer's Disease

Curiously, there was not conclusive evidence in favour of the "magnocellular deficit hypothesis" till now, neither of a damage of the retinocalcarine pathway associated with AD (Jacob et al., 2002). For example, Rizzo et al. argued that visual impairment in AD is totally due to dysfunction in the associative cortices, basing their theory on normality of VEPs, full-field ERG and cortical flicker fusion threshold in AD patients (Rizzo et al., 1992; Rizzo et al., 2000). On the other hand, the sensory deficits can be hidden and frequently masquerade as higher order deficits.

Tippett et al. investigated whether high-level visual processing are primary involved in mild-to-moderate AD, by using items of the Birmingham Object Recognition Battery.

These tests are based on the recognition of a target when some components has been obscured by rotating images, or on the identification of a "real" animal compared to a "not real" one (i.e. a chicken versus an animal made-up by putting a donkey's head on a chicken's body). Since AD patients were able to distinguish the real animals and name them, they concluded that weakened or distorted visual inputs come from basic shape processing areas only, even if face processing is also impaired in AD patients.

These results are consistent with the view that face recognition relies on neural representations relatively independent from those implicated in object processing. These data seem to indicate two distinct pathways of visual processing altered in mild-to-moderate AD, basic shape perception and face processing. To rule out a primary, high-order visual impairment in AD it's worth considering that (1) there is no relation between visual task performance and MMSE score (Mini-Mental State Examination) and (2) truly segregated and symmetrical opponent-color systems do not exist in the cortex, where both luminance information and chromatic contrasts are simultaneously processed to detect spatial patterns (Regan, 1989).

Another interesting issue is whether the two hemispheres are asymmetrically involved in AD patients: in fact, the right hemisphere is dominant for rod-mediated scotopico behavior, whereas the left one may be dominant for cone-mediated photopic behavior (Braun et al., 1998).

Making the Difference Between Central and Peripheral Visual Involvement in Alzheimer's Disease

In the past, the reason for a caution interpretation of previously reported evidences is that there are many contradictory signs of a specific visual involvement: shrinkage of both P and M ganglion cells in the retina, thinning of the nerve fiber layer (Berisha et al., 2007), as well as pathology in both the magno- and the parvocellular layers of lateral geniculate nucleus (LGN), without any definitive conclusion on the selective vulnerability of a visual subsystem. Some authors concluded that the unspecific alterations in second-order neurons pool reflects an initial age-dependent photoreceptors dysfunctions (Gresh et al., 2003). Since age-dependent modifications were substantially the same for sensitivity to luminance and colour contrast (Ruddock, 1965; Suzuki, 2006), it has been argued that they all arise at a peripheral level, with obvious reference to senile miosis, increased intraocular light scatter, decreased retinal blood flow in narrow veins or opacification of the ocular media (Fiorentini et al., 1996), promoted by Aβ proteins aggregation. Some authors have also described a disease-related enlargement of the optic nerve head cupping as well as a marked thinning of neuroretinal rim (Berisha et al., 2007). For instance, it cannot be excluded that the outer retina may show some signs of impairment in AD patients: in fact, age-dependent morphological alterations in second-order retinal neurons is commonly accompanied by dendrites loss, redistribution of glutamate receptors and simplification of horizontal cells network (Strettoi et al., 2002; Terzibasi et al., 2009). These all processes are characterized by a clear spatial gradient, increasing in number from the centre to the periphery of the retina. However, it's worth remembering that compensatory remodeling, in relation to gradual increase in both ectopic synapses and collateral sprouting, follows a similar trend from the periphery, where magnocellular pathway arises, to foveal and parafoveal areas (Terzibasi et al., 2009).

Besides, it is likely that retinal ganglion cell loss may be partially secondary to retrograde axonal degeneration too, since there's a greater degeneration in the posterior optic nerve (Hinton et al., 1986). Taken together, these evidences play against a peripheral source of visual impairment in AD, consistent with the findings that AD particularly affects either cortico-cortical projection neurons (Hof et al., 1990; Kavcic et al., 2006) or geniculo-calcarine processing.

Conclusions

In conclusion our data showed evident abnormalities both in latency and amplitude of LumPERGs, and no significant changes in ChPERGs, in AD patients. Moreover, starting from clinical aspects and neuropathological changes, with focus on the visual system and the subsystem organization of visual pathways, we brought a further evidence of involvement of the magnocellular stream or, in cortex, of the dorsal processing stream, supporting a formative theory that propose exceptional vulnerability of functions associated with the magnocellular pathway in AD. In fact, even if in a relatively small samples of patients, our electrophysiological findings suggest that M-stream could be the best candidate to explain impairments of visual function in this disease. We believe that further studies should be conducted with larger sample sizes to confirm these results and expanded to include other specific forms of vision testing; it is also desirable that better understanding of vision-related magnocellular impairment could guide interventions to improve functional capacity in patients with dementia.

References

Alladi S, Xuereb J, Bak T, Nestor P, Knibb J, Patterson K, Hodges JR (2007) Focal cortical presentations of Alzheimer's disease. *Brain* 130:2636-2645.

Arancio O, Zhang HP, Chen X, Lin C, Trinchese F, Puzzo D, Liu S, Hegde A, Yan SF, Stern A, Luddy JS, Lue LF, Walker DG, Roher A, Buttini M, Mucke L, Li W, Schmidt AM, Kindy M, Hyslop PA, Stern DM, Du Yan SS (2004) RAGE potentiates Abeta-induced perturbation of neuronal function in transgenic mice. *EMBO J* 23:4096-4105.

Berisha F, Feke GT, Trempe CL, McMeel JW, Schepens CL (2007) Retinal abnormalities in early Alzheimer's disease. *Invest Ophthalmol Vis Sci* 48:2285-2289.

Blanks JC, Hinton DR, Sadun AA, Miller CA (1989) Retinal ganglion cell degeneration in Alzheimer's disease. *Brain Res* 501:364-372.

Braun CM, Achim A, Charron JF, Cote A (1998) Dissociation of hemispheric exploitation of rods and cones for simple detection. *Am J Psychol* 111:241-263.

Brodie EE AD, Brooks DN, McCulloch J, Foulds WS. (1992) Flash and pattern reversal visual evoked responses in normal and demented elderly. *Cortex* 28:289-293.

Bruban J, Glotin AL, Dinet V, Chalour N, Sennlaub F, Jonet L, An N, Faussat AM, Mascarelli F (2009) Amyloid-beta(1-42) alters structure and function of retinal pigmented epithelial cells. *Aging Cell* 8:162-177.

Cronin-Golomb A, Hof PR (2004) *Vision in Alzheimer's disease*. S. Karger AG, Basel (Switzerland).

Cronin-Golomb A, Rizzo JF, Corkin S, Growdon JH (1991) Visual function in Alzheimer's disease and normal aging. *Ann N Y Acad Sci* 640:28-35.

Crum RM, Anthony JC, Bassett SS, Folstein MF (1993) Population-based norms for the Mini-Mental State Examination by age and educational level. *JAMA* 269:2386-2391.

Dacey DM, Lee BB (1994) The 'blue-on' opponent pathway in primate retina originates from a distinct bistratified ganglion cell type. *Nature* 367:731-735.

De Monasterio FM, Gouras P (1975) Functional properties of ganglion cells of the rhesus monkey retina. *J Physiol* 251:167-195.

Dentchev T, Milam AH, Lee VM, Trojanowski JQ, Dunaief JL (2003) Amyloid-beta is found in drusen from some age-related macular degeneration retinas, but not in drusen from normal retinas. *Mol Vis* 9:184-190.

Di Russo F, Spinelli D (1999) Spatial attention has different effects on the magno- and parvocellular pathways. *NeuroReport* 10:2755-2762.

Dreher B, Fukada Y, Rodieck RW (1976) Identification, classification and anatomical segregation of cells with X-like and Y-like properties in the lateral geniculate nucleus of old-world primates. *J Physiol* 258:433-452.

Duffy CJ, Tetewsky SJ, O'Brien H (2000) Cortical motion blindness in visuospatial AD. *Neurobiol Aging* 21:867-869; discussion 875-867.

Dutescu RM, Li QX, Crowston J, Masters CL, Baird PN, Culvenor JG (2009) Amyloid precursor protein processing and retinal pathology in mouse models of Alzheimer's disease. *Graefes Arch Clin Exp Ophthalmol* 247:1213-1221.

Engel S, Zhang X, Wandell B (1997) Colour tuning in human visual cortex measured with functional magnetic resonance imaging. *Nature* 388:68-71.

Erkinjuntti T, Ketonen L, Sulkava R, Sipponen J, Vuorialho M, Iivanainen M (1987) Do white matter changes on MRI and CT differentiate vascular dementia from Alzheimer's disease? *J Neurol Neurosurg Psychiatry* 50:37-42.

Fiorentini A PV, Morrone MC, Burr DC (1996) Visual ageing: unspecific decline of the responses to luminance and colour. *Vision Res* 36:3557–3356.

Gandy S (2005) The role of cerebral amyloid beta accumulation in common forms of Alzheimer disease. *J Clin Invest* 115:1121-1129.

Gilmore GC WH, Naylor LA, Koss E. (1994) Motion perception and Alzheimer's disease. *J Gerontol* 49:P52-57.

Gomez-Isla T, Price JL, McKeel DW, Jr., Morris JC, Growdon JH, Hyman BT (1996) Profound loss of layer II entorhinal cortex neurons occurs in very mild Alzheimer's disease. *J Neurosci* 16:4491-4500.

Gresh J, Goletz PW, Crouch RK, Rohrer B (2003) Structure-function analysis of rods and cones in juvenile, adult, and aged C57bl/6 and Balb/c mice. *Vis Neurosci* 20:211-220.

Hasselmo ME, Giocomo LM (2006) Cholinergic modulation of cortical function. *J Mol Neurosci* 30:133-135.

Hinton DR, Sadun AA, Blanks JC, Miller CA (1986) Optic-nerve degeneration in Alzheimer's disease. *N Engl J Med* 315:485-487.

Hof PR, Morrison JH (1990) Quantitative analysis of a vulnerable subset of pyramidal neurons in Alzheimer's disease: II. Primary and secondary visual cortex. *J Comp Neurol* 301:55-64.

Hof PR, Bouras C, Constantinidis J, Morrison JH (1990) Selective disconnection of specific visual association pathways in cases of Alzheimer's disease presenting with Balint's syndrome. *J Neuropathol Exp Neurol* 49:168-184.

Hsia AY, Masliah E, McConlogue L, Yu GQ, Tatsuno G, Hu K, Kholodenko D, Malenka RC, Nicoll RA, Mucke L (1999) Plaque-independent disruption of neural circuits in Alzheimer's disease mouse models. *Proc Natl Acad Sci U S A* 96:3228-3233.

Hsiao K, Chapman P, Nilsen S, Eckman C, Harigaya Y, Younkin S, Yang F, Cole G (1996) Correlative memory deficits, Abeta elevation, and amyloid plaques in transgenic mice. *Science* 274:99-102.

Hyman BT, Van Hoesen GW, Damasio AR, Barnes CL (1984) Alzheimer's disease: cell-specific pathology isolates the hippocampal formation. *Science* 225:1168-1170.

Jacob B, Hache JC, Pasquier F (2002) [Dysfunction of the magnocellular pathway in Alzheimer's disease]. *Rev Neurol* (Paris) 158:555-564.

Jacobsen JS, Wu CC, Redwine JM, Comery TA, Arias R, Bowlby M, Martone R, Morrison JH, Pangalos MN, Reinhart PH, Bloom FE (2006) Early-onset behavioral and synaptic deficits in a mouse model of Alzheimer's disease. *Proc Natl Acad Sci U S A* 103:5161-5166.

Kavcic V, Fernandez R, Logan D, Duffy CJ (2006) Neurophysiological and perceptual correlates of navigational impairment in Alzheimer's disease. *Brain* 129:736-746.

Lennie P, Krauskopf J, Sclar G (1990) Chromatic mechanisms in striate cortex of macaque. *J Neurosci* 10:649-669.

McKhnann G, Drachman D, Folstein M, Katzman R, Price D, Stadlan EM (1984): Clinical diagnosis of Alzheimer's disease: Report of the NINCDS-ADRDA work group under the auspices of Department of Health and Human Services Task Force on Alzheimer's disease. *Neurology*, 34: 939-944.

Mendez MF, Tomsak RL, Remler B (1990) Disorders of the visual system in Alzheimer's disease. *J Clin Neuroophthalmol* 10:62-69.

Merigan WH, Maunsell JH (1993) How parallel are the primate visual pathways? *Annu Rev Neurosci* 16:369-402.

Moore NC (1997) Visual evoked responses in Alzheimer's disease: a review. *Clin Electroencephalogr* 28:137-142.

Mullen KT (1985) The contrast sensitivity of human colour vision to red-green and blue-yellow chromatic gratings. *J. Physiol.* 359, 381-400.

Ng SY, Villemagne VL, Masters CL, Rowe CC (2007) Evaluating atypical dementia syndromes using positron emission tomography with carbon 11 labeled Pittsburgh Compound B. *Arch Neurol* 64:1140-1144.

Origlia N, Capsoni S, Cattaneo A, Fang F, Arancio O, Yan SD, Domenici L (2009) Abeta-dependent Inhibition of LTP in different intracortical circuits of the visual cortex: the role of RAGE. *J Alzheimers Dis* 17:59-68.

Porciatti V, Sartucci F (1996) Retinal and cortical evoked responses to chromatic contrast stimuli. Specific losses in both eyes of patients with multiple sclerosis and unilateral optic neuritis. *Brain* 119 (Pt 3):723-740.

Porciatti V, Sartucci F (1999) Normative data for onset VEPs to red-green and blue-yellow chromatic contrast. *Clin Neurophysiol* 110:772-781.

Redwine JM, Kosofsky B, Jacobs RE, Games D, Reilly JF, Morrison JH, Young WG, Bloom FE (2003) Dentate gyrus volume is reduced before onset of plaque formation in PDAPP mice: a magnetic resonance microscopy and stereologic analysis. *Proc Natl Acad Sci U S A* 100:1381-1386.

Regan D (1989) *Human brain electrophysiology : evoked potentials and evoked magnetic fields in science and medicine.* New York: Elsevier.

Rizzo JF, 3rd, Cronin-Golomb A, Growdon JH, Corkin S, Rosen TJ, Sandberg MA, Chiappa KH, Lessell S (1992) Retinocalcarine function in Alzheimer's disease. A clinical and electrophysiological study. *Arch Neurol* 49:93-101.

Rizzo M, Anderson SW, Dawson J, Nawrot M (2000) Vision and cognition in Alzheimer's disease. *Neuropsychologia* 38:1157-1169.

Ruddock K (1965) The effect of age upon colour vision. II. Changes with age in light transmission of the ocular media. *Vision Res* 5:47-58.

Sartucci F, Borghetti D, Bocci T, Murri L, Orsini P, Porciatti V, Origlia N, Domenici L (2010): Dysfunction of the magnocellular stream in Alzheimer's disease evaluated by pattern electroretinograms and visual evoked potentials. *Brain Res Bull.,* 82 (3-4): 169-76.

Scheltens P, Kittner B (2000) Preliminary results from an MRI/CT-based database for vascular dementia and Alzheimer's disease. *Ann N Y Acad Sci* 903:542-546.

Selkoe DJ (2002) Alzheimer's disease is a synaptic failure. *Science* 298:789-791.

Shapley R (1990) Visual sensitivity and parallel retinocortical channels. *Annu Rev Psychol* 41:635-658.

Strettoi E, Porciatti V, Falsini B, Pignatelli V, Rossi C (2002) Morphological and functional abnormalities in the inner retina of the rd/rd mouse. *J Neurosci* 22:5492-5504.

Stromer T, Serpell LC (2005) Structure and morphology of the Alzheimer's amyloid fibril. *Microsc Res Tech* 67:210-217.

Suzuki TA QY, Sakuragawa S, Tamura H, Okajima K. (2006) Age-related changes of reaction time and p300 for low-contrast color stimuli: Effects of yellowing of the aging human lens. *J Physiol Anthropol* 25:179-187.

Terzibasi E, Calamusa M, Novelli E, Domenici L, Strettoi E, Cellerino A (2009) Age-dependent remodelling of retinal circuitry. *Neurobiol Aging* 30:819-828.

Tierney MC, Fisher RH, Lewis AJ, Zorzitto ML, Snow WG, Reid DW, Nieuwstraten P (1988) The NINCDS-ADRDA Work Group criteria for the clinical diagnosis of probable Alzheimer's disease: a clinicopathologic study of 57 cases. *Neurology* 38:359-364.

Tippett LJ, Blackwood K, Farah MJ (2003) Visual object and face processing in mild-to-moderate Alzheimer's disease: from segmentation to imagination. *Neuropsychologia* 41 (4): 453-68.

Tognoni G, Ceravolo R, Nucciarone B, Bianchi F, Dell'Agnello G, Ghicopulos I, Siciliano G, Murri L (2005) From mild cognitive impairment to dementia: a prevalence study in a district of Tuscany, Italy. *Acta Neurol Scand* 112:65-71.

Valenti D (2004) The anterior visual system and circadian function with reference to Alzheimer's Disease. In: Cronin-Golomb & Hof PR (eds): *Vision in Alzheimer's disease*, S. Karger AG, Basel (Switzerland), 1-29.

Van Essen DC, Gallant JL (1994) Neural mechanisms of form and motion processing in the primate visual system. *Neuron* 13:1-10.

Von Gunten A, Giannakopoulos P, Bouras C, Hof PR (2004) Neuropathological changes in visuospatial systems in Alzheimer's disease. In: Cronin-Golomb & Hof PR (eds): *Vision in Alzheimer's disease,* S. Karger AG, Basel (Switzerland), 1-29.

In: Alzheimer's Diagnosis
Editor: Charles E. Ronson, pp. 43-59

ISBN: 978-1-61209-846-3
©2011 Nova Science Publishers, Inc.

Chapter III

Alzheimer's Disease Diagnosis: A New Approach

Ana Valverde and Sónia Costa

Neurology Department, Hospital Fernando Fonseca, Lisbon. Portugal

Abstract

Clinical neuroscience has an increasing need for new methods to identify the earliest features of neurodegenerative disorders such as Alzheimer's disease (AD) and other dementias. This growing interest in the pre-dementia phase of these conditions aims to identify them before functional impairment is evident. Ideally before this phase, treatment of the underlying disease would postpone its process. A variety of clinical, imaging and laboratory methods has emerged during the last decade to allow more accurate diagnosis of AD. A review of these new markers will be made with reference to the new diagnostic criteria proposed by the International Working Group in Alzheimer's disease.

Introduction

Alzheimer's disease (AD) is the most common cause of dementia [1]. It's a complex neurodegenerative condition which has become a major public health problem because of its increasing prevalence, long duration and high cost of care.

As recently as two or three decades ago, a compartmentalied model of Alzheimer's disease was accepted. According to this model, people either had AD pathological changes, in which case they had dementia, or they did not have such changes and were cognitively normal [2]. This view has changed, and today we know that pathological changes start in the medial temporal lobe and precede the first dementia symptoms by 10 years or more [3,4].

On the other hand, historically, there has been a dichotomy in the use of AD to refer to either the clinical or the neuropathological entity, that caused confusion, particularly in light of repeated reports that pathological changes can exist in elderly persons without the concomitant clinical manifestations of AD [5,6].

The incremental growth of scientific knowledge around the pathogenic events and course of AD has significantly advanced our view of the disease and its defining boundaries.

In 2007, the International Working Group for New Research Criteria for the Diagnosis of AD proposed a new diagnostic framework [7] to move beyond the "classical" criteria from the National Institute of Neurological and Communicative Disorders and Stroke-Alzheimer's Disease and Related Disorders Association (NINCDS-ADRDA) criteria [8]. According to these criteria, AD diagnosis is made when there is both clinical evidence of the disease phenotype and in-vivo biological evidence of AD pathology. With this algorithm, diagnosis could be done even in the earliest stages with a reasonable level of accuracy. Conditions within the new research criteria include asymptomatic patients with positive biomarkers for AD pathology, clinically symptomatic individuals without evidence of biomarker findings and those with atypical features (non-amnestic focal-cortical syndromes, such as progressive non-fluent logopenic aphasia [9] and posterior cortical atrophy [10]) confirmed pathologically as being AD. This proposal was a stimulating scientific advance but had some caveats: it did not address AD- related stages with no clinicobiological duality.

Recently, a new paper was developed by the International Working Group to provide a companion lexicon wherein the different entities and concepts related to AD are defined and updated, as a point of reference for the clinical and research communities. Hence, AD would be considered as a clinical and symptomatic entity that encompasses both pre-dementia and dementia phases [11].

Multi-Modal Techniques for Diagnosis of AD

Classic Assessment of AD Dementia

Obtaining a detailed history from the patient and a reliable caregiver is of primary importance in diagnosing AD. The most common presenting symptom is insidious episodic memory impairment, often involving names of persons or objects. Visuospatial deficits are often recognized when patients become lost or disoriented while navigating. Misplacing of personal objects with increasing frequency, may also reveal a visual memory deficit. Reduced spontaneous verbal output often accompanies early memory symptoms, but many patients develop other language deficits, including anomia and non-fluency with prominent word-finding problems, hesitancy and occasional paraphasic errors. Grammar and syntax may also become progressive less complex.

Other cognitive symptoms such as executive dysfunction and apraxia, occur more often in the moderate or late stages. Neuropsychiatric symptoms such as apathy, depression and agitation are reported in up to 80% of patients with AD, and become more common as the illness progresses.

These concerns reflect the characteristic spread of AD pathology along the different cortical areas.

The initial presentation can also be atypical with non-amnestic focal cortical cognitive symptoms [10].

Formal cognitive testing can aid to diagnose AD , and is particularly useful for clinical situations in which cognitive symptoms and signs are subtle or confounded by other medical factors such as depression. A variety of neuropsychological tests can be used to accurately assess the different cognitive domains [12]. Using an episodic memory test that assesses response to cueing, AD has been identified in patients two years before the dementia phase with a high specificity [13]. Serial neuropsychological evaluations are also very useful for tracking the progress of an individual over time relative to an established baseline.

In 2001, the American Academy of Neurology updated guidelines for dementia diagnosis, regarding the usefulness of laboratory testing in the initial clinical assessment using an evidence-based approach [14]. These guidelines recommended screening for depression, hypothyroidism and vitamin B12 deficiency as potentially treatable causes of cognitive impairment, as well as neuroimaging as part of an initial evaluation for possible dementia. Structural neuroimaging with MRI or non-contrast CT scan allowed the clinician to exclude structural pathology, including neoplasms, cerebrovascular lesions and hydrocephalus, and confirming the typical changes associated with AD.

Several other laboratory tests such as syphilis screening might be recommended depending on the clinical scenario.

Electroencephalogram (EEG), usually not recommended for routine use, being often normal in AD, might be useful in distinguishing dementia from delirium and for diagnosing seizures. Seizures may be present in up to 17% of AD cases and up to 6% at the time of diagnosis

To address the diagnostic uncertainty, the 1984 NINCDS-ADRDA criteria stipulated that AD diagnosis during life could only be "probable", whereas a "definite" diagnosis required post-mortem histopathological confirmation (Table 1) [8].

Table 1.

NINCDS-ADRDA criteria for a clinical diagnosis of probable Alzheimer's Disease (from MacKhann G *et al.*, 1984)
☉1 Memory impairment
•2 One or more impairments in the cognitive domains:
1.   Language (aphasia)
2.   Motor activities (apraxia)
3.   Visual perception (agnosia)
4.   Executive function (executive dysfunction)
•1 Impaired social or occupational function
•2 Gradual onset, gradual progression
•3 No other CSN disease/systemic disorders known to cause cognitive impairment

However, there were some drawbacks: These clinical criteria largely depends on exclusion of other dementia, and even in patients followed up clinically for several years, the diagnostic accuracy is relatively low, with a specificity of around 70% and a sensitivity of 80% [14]

Additionally, the term AD was also used to refer to the pathological process defined by specific neuronal lesions including senile plaques and neurofibrillary tangles, associated with neuronal loss, synaptic loss and frequently with cerebral amyloid angiopathy [15]. This pathological process might or might not become symptomatic during life [16, 17]. Because of a lack of a clear understanding of the relation between the neuropathological pattern and its clinical occurrence, a division between clinical expression and underlying pathology was recently proposed [11].

New Research Criteria for the Diagnosis of AD: An Attempt to Improve Clinical Diagnosis Accuracy

A growing body of evidence supports today the independence of AD onset from cognitive status. The hallmark histopathological features, amyloid plaques and neurofibrillary tangles (NFT) actually define but do not fully represent the disease process. It also involves inflammation, neuronal, axonal and synaptic loss. The onset of very mild dementia is correlated best with significant synaptic and neuronal loss [18]. During "pre-clinical" AD, plaques and subsequently NFT accumulate. It lasts about 10-15 years until synaptic and neuronal loss manifest as cognitive decline [3]. This concept fits with genetic, biochemical and animal model data which demonstrate that the aggregation of amyloid β (Aβ) peptide plays a role in the pre-clinical phase of AD, and that tau aggregation, which occurs later, drives neurodegeneration just prior and during clinical phase [19]. Over the past two decades, it became possible to identify in-vivo evidence of the specific neuropathology of AD [20, 21].There are two broad categories of biomarkers: biochemical and neuroimaging. Both are very highly correlated with AD neuropathological lesions [22-25]. These biomarkers can also be divided into pathophysiological and topographical markers (table 2).

Table 2.

Pathophysiological biomarkers:
   ▪🗀   CSF amyloid β.
     ▪🗎 CSF total tau, phospho tau.
     ▪🗎 PET amyloid tracer uptake.
Topographical biomarkers:
   ▪🗀   Fluorodeoxyglucose PET.
     ▪🗎 Structural MRI: Medial Temporal Atrophy.

Pathophysiological markers correspond to the two aetiological degenerative processes that characterise AD pathology: the amyloidosis path to neuritic plaques and the tauopathy path to NFT [15]. They include CSF measures of reduced concentrations of amyloid β, increased total tau, and increased phospho-tau [22,23,25,26] and amyloid PET scanning with Pittsburgh compound B (PiB) [24,27]or other radioligands. Topographical markers are used to assess the less specific brain changes that correlate with the regional distribution of Alzheimer's pathology and include medial temporal lobe atrophy [28, 29] and reduced glucose metabolism in temporo-parietal regions on fluorodeoxyglucose PET [30]. Understanding the timing of pathological events, allows us to know that pathophysiological changes precede the topographical ones associated with neurodegeneration [31]. According to this sequence of events, pathophysiological markers could have a diagnostic use at all disease stages, including the pre-clinical stage, whereas topographical markers would be more useful closer to the time when the cognitive symptoms are present. Nevertheless, regional hypometabolism with fluorodeoxyglucose PET has been described in asymptomatic adults with genetic susceptibility for AD [32,33].

Biochemical Biomarkers

The search for biochemical markers of AD in body fluids began with the "Consensus Report of the Working Group on Molecular and Biochemical Markers of Alzheimer's Disease" published in 1998 [34]. The working group provided guidelines for an ideal AD biomarker: it should detect a fundamental feature of the neuropathology and be validated in neuropathologically confirmed cases with a sensitivity of more than 80% for distinguishing other dementias. Other desirable features included being technically reliable and reproductible, non-invasive, simple to perform and inexpensive.

The cerebrospinal fluid (CSF) represents the most direct and convenient means to study the biochemical changes occurring in the central nervous system (CNS). The major protein constituents of AD pathology, beta-amyloid peptide 42 (Aβ42), tau protein and phosphorylated tau protein 181 (p-tau181p) [35] closest fulfilled the criteria described above.

Aβ is a secreted peptide of unknown physiological function, cleaved from the amyloid precursor protein (APP) by the sequential activities of beta and gamma secretase enzymes. Most of this peptide is produced in the brain and effluxes into CSF, appearing at relatively high levels. It has multiple forms according to amino acids quantity. Among these, Aβ42 appears to be essential for initiating Aβ aggregation. Its paper is central to AD amyloid cascade hypothesis, and in this way, it serves as a very useful biomarker [19]. As a result from the deposition of the peptide in plaques, avoiding its transit into the CSF, CSF Aβ42 is significantly reduced in AD subjects [36]. In the past 11 years, scores of studies have been published from investigators world-wide, reporting that the formula of low Aβ42 level and high tau and p-tau 181 levels denoted AD with high sensibility and specificity [34].

Tau is a cytosolic neuron protein, whose function apparently is to maintain microtubule stability within the axon. This function is regulated principally by serine and threonine residues phosphorylation. In AD, hyperphosphorylated tau usually fills the dystrophic neurites or neuritis plaques, and is the component of the paired helical filaments that constitute NFT. The mechanism to appear in the CSF is not well known, but it's widely assumed that the major sources of CSF tau and phosphorylated tau are neuronal injury, death and NFT [37].

CSF Aβ and tau measurements met the first and most important criterion of reflecting an important neuropathologic feature of AD. What is measured in CSF reflects the biochemical composition of the anatomic lesions: levels of Aβ42 inversely correlate with the total Aβ load in the brain and tau protein levels directly with the presence of neocortical neurofibrillary tangles in an autopsy-confirmed series of cases [36]. The sensitivity of the test for distinguishing AD from healthy controls was also proved high: 90% in those with AD, 72% in those with mild cognitive impairment (MCI) and 36% in controls, with an overall diagnostic specificity of 64% [38]. Furthermore, the AD CSF signature correctly identified 100% of MCI cases that progressed to AD within 5 years [38], so it would be a possible predictive value in detecting AD in advance of clinical signs and symptoms.

Additionally, CSF biomarkers may be able to identify AD pathology in atypical focal cortical presentations of AD, such as Posterior Cortical Atrophy (PCA) and Logopenic Progressive Primary Aphasia (PPA) [10,39], and may improve the in vivo differential diagnosis between AD and both Frontotemporal Dementia (FTD) and Semantic Dementia (SD) , which have different neuropathological causes [40].

The pathology of AD involves many other processes: microglial activation, inflammation, oxidative processes, and finally, loss of synapses and neuronal dying. Each of these changes may also serve for searching other fluid biomarkers that may complement or improve the utility of CSF Aβ42 and tau [41].

Neuroimaging Biomarkers

Aβ and Tau Images

Until recently, antemortem examination of the pathological changes was impossible. Within the last decade, a number of radiological contrast compounds have been developed that specifically bind and highlight pathological structures in the CNS [42].

Of the amyloid-binding compounds, ^{11}C-PiB, short for "Pittsburgh Compound-B", has been extensively studied and applied in AD research. The uptake of PiB can be measured by positron emission tomography (PET). In AD, an increased retention of PiB shows a specific pattern that is restricted to brain regions typically associated with amyloid deposition [27]. PiB-PET uptake correlates inversely with CSF Aβ42 levels, consisting of the idea that soluble Aβ42 is retained in the brain once plaques are formed [20]. Moreover, high cortical binding values for PiB-PET are predictive of cognitive decline and AD development in cognitive, normal elderly subjects [42].

Other PET labelling agents have been developed to image inflammation, but larger studies will be needed to improve the molecular imaging.

Measures pf Synaptic Activity - Functional MRI (fMRI)

Neurons of the medial temporal lobes and hippocampus are particularly susceptible to loss in AD, and their loss appears to coincide with the onset of clinically significant cognitive impairment. Accordingly, the medial temporal lobe system shows hypoactivation in the clinical stages of AD, and interestingly, the same structures show hyperactivaton in pre-dementia phases in an attempt to compensate for functional deficits [43]. Other cortical regions that also have amyloid deposition (e.g. posterior cingulate, precuneus, temporo-parietal and medial frontal), show the same changes even in pre-clinical phases.

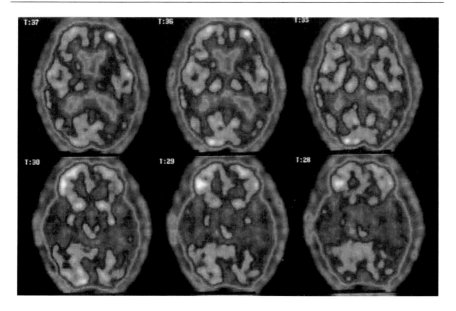

Figure 1.

Glucose-Metabolism Imaging

As might be expected for brain regions that display atrophy and neuronal loss, these cortical regions also show evidence of reduced glucose metabolism in AD, as measured by fluoro-deoxyglucose (FDG-PET) [44] (Figure 1). Although its accuracy has not been thoroughly compared to other biomarkers assessed in the same subjects, FDG-PET has been reported to predict conversion to AD [45], and correlates with the level of cognitive impairment [46].

Structural Neuroimaging

The characteristic patterns of cortical and hippocampal atrophy in advanced AD are well known but difficult to quantify at post-mortem examination (Figure 2). In early AD stages, difficulty increases because it resembles the volume commonly observed among elderly persons without neurodegeneration.

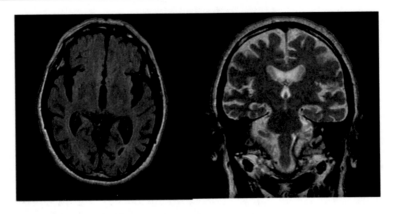

Figure 2.

Table 3.

Proposed (research) diagnosis criteria for AD (from Dubois B *et al.* 2007) Probable AD: A plus one or more supportive features B, C, D, or E
Core diagnostic criteria

A. Presence of an early and significant episodic memory impairment that includes the following features:
  • Gradual and progressive change in memory function reported by patients or informants over more than 6 months.
  • Objective evidence of significantly impaired episodic memory on testing: this generally consists of recall deficit that does not improve significantly or does not normalize with cueing or recognition testing and after effective encoding of information has been previously controlled
  • The episodic memory impairment can be isolated or associated with other cognitive changes at the onset of AD or as AD advances
B. *Supportive features*
C. Presence of medial temporal lobe atrophy
  • Volume loss of hippocampi, entorhinal cortex, amygdala evidenced on MRI with qualitative ratings using visual scoring (referenced to well-characterized population with age norms) or quantitative volumetry of regions of interest (referenced to well- characterized population with age norms)
D. Abnormal cerebrospinal fluid biomarker
  • Low amyloid β1–42 concentrations, increased total tau concentrations, or increased phospho-tau concentrations, or combinations of the three

- Other well-validated markers to be discovered in the future
E. Specific pattern on functional neuroimaging with PET
- Reduced glucose metabolism in bilateral temporal parietal regions
- Other well-validated ligands, including those that foreseeably will emerge, such as Pittsburg compound B or FDDNP
F. Proven AD autosomal dominant mutation within the immediate family

Exclusion criteria
History
- Sudden onset
- Early occurrence of the following symptoms: gait disturbances, seizures, behavioral changes

Clinical features
- Focal neurological features including hemiparesis, sensory loss, visual field deficits
- Early extrapyramidal signs

Other medical disorders severe enough to account for memory and related symptoms
- Non-AD dementia
- Major depression
- Cerebrovascular disease
- Toxic and metabolic abnormalities, all of which may require specific investigations
MRI FLAIR or T2 signal abnormalities in the medial temporal lobe that are consistent with infectious or vascular insults

Criteria for definite AD
AD is considered definite if the following are present:
- Both clinical and histopathological (brain biopsy or autopsy) evidence of the disease, as required by the NIA-Reagan criteria for the post-mortem diagnosis of AD; criteria must both be present139
- • Both clinical and genetic evidence (mutation on chromosome 1, 14, or 21) of AD; criteria must both be present

With high resolution MRI, such subtle differences may be distinguished, especially when applied longitudinally and global atrophy rates are calculated [47]. MRI and PET topographical markers have been shown to correlate consistently with disease severity [48]. Some of the biomarkers have greater specificity for Alzheimer's pathology within a particular context: while medial temporal lobe atrophy can occur in non-AD dementias [49], a low CSF Aβ42 or a positive amyloid result on PET imaging might be more specific for the amyloidosis associated with AD. Revision of research criteria for the diagnosis of AD that includes abnormal biomarkers has been proposed (table 3) [7].

Thereby, clinical and in-vivo manifestations of the disease can now be integrated into the diagnosis, and this no longer needs to be anchored to a dementia syndrome as it is done so far.

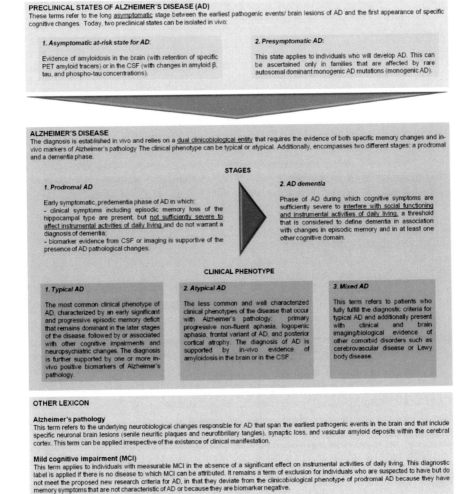

PRECLINICAL STATES OF ALZHEIMER'S DISEASE (AD)
These terms refer to the long asymptomatic stage between the earliest pathogenic events/ brain lesions of AD and the first appearance of specific cognitive changes. Today, two preclinical states can be isolated in vivo:

1. Asymptomatic at-risk state for AD:

Evidence of amyloidosis in the brain (with retention of specific PET amyloid tracers) or in the CSF (with changes in amyloid β, tau, and phospho-tau concentrations).

2. Presymptomatic AD:

This state applies to individuals who will develop AD. This can be ascertained only in families that are affected by rare autosomal dominant monogenic AD mutations (monogenic AD).

ALZHEIMER'S DISEASE
The diagnosis is established in vivo and relies on a dual clinicobiological entity that requires the evidence of both specific memory changes and in-vivo markers of Alzheimer's pathology The clinical phenotype can be typical or atypical. Additionally, encompasses two different stages: a prodromal and a dementia phase.

STAGES

1. Prodromal AD

Early symptomatic, predementia phase of AD in which:
- clinical symptoms including episodic memory loss of the hippocampal type are present, but not sufficiently severe to affect instrumental activities of daily living and do not warrant a diagnosis of dementia;
- biomarker evidence from CSF or imaging is supportive of the presence of AD pathological changes.

2. AD dementia

Phase of AD during which cognitive symptoms are sufficiently severe to interfere with social functioning and instrumental activities of daily living, a threshold that is considered to define dementia in association with changes in episodic memory and in at least one other cognitive domain.

CLINICAL PHENOTYPE

1. Typical AD

The most common clinical phenotype of AD, characterized by an early significant and progressive episodic memory deficit that remains dominant in the later stages of the disease, followed by or associated with other cognitive impairments and neuropsychiatric changes. The diagnosis is further supported by one or more in-vivo positive biomarkers of Alzheimer's pathology.

2. Atypical AD

The less common and well characterized clinical phenotypes of the disease that occur with Alzheimer's pathology: primary progressive non-fluent aphasia, logopenic aphasia, frontal variant of AD, and posterior cortical atrophy. The diagnosis of AD is supported by in-vivo evidence of amyloidosis in the brain or in the CSF.

3. Mixed AD

This term refers to patients who fully fulfill the diagnostic criteria for typical AD and additionally present with clinical and brain imaging/biological evidence of other comorbid disorders such as cerebrovascular disease or Lewy body disease.

OTHER LEXICON

Alzheimer's pathology
This term refers to the underlying neurobiological changes responsible for AD that span the earliest pathogenic events in the brain and that include specific neuronal brain lesions (senile neuritic plaques and neurofibrillary tangles), synaptic loss, and vascular amyloid deposits within the cerebral cortex. This term can be applied irrespective of the existence of clinical manifestation.

Mild cognitive impairment (MCI)
This term applies to individuals with measurable MCI in the absence of a significant effect on instrumental activities of daily living. This diagnostic label is applied if there is no disease to which MCI can be attributed. It remains a term of exclusion for individuals who are suspected to have but do not meet the proposed new research criteria for AD, in that they deviate from the clinicobiological phenotype of prodromal AD because they have memory symptoms that are not characteristic of AD or because they are biomarker negative.

Figure 3.

According to these guidelines, AD is defined in vivo with a gradual, slowly progressive episodic memory impairment that is documented on formal testing, and supportive biomarkers are required that indicate the pathophysiology or the topography of Alzheimer's pathology. Earlier disease recognition is possible and the borders between clinical and pre-clinical stages of AD might shift. Within this algorithm, the designation of "probable" and "possible" is changed by "typical" and "atypical" AD because of the use of reliable biomarkers (Figure 3). A restatement of the definition of AD and related stages is in process [11].

On the basis of this novel diagnostic approach, the term "Alzheimer's disease" has been proposed to be used to the in-vivo clinicobiological expression of the disease as it should encompass the whole spectrum of its clinical course [11]. Problems such as "atypical Alzheimer's disease" (non-amnestic focal cortical syndromes) and "mixed Alzheimer's disease" (co-ocurrence of Alzheimer's pathology and comorbid disorders: cerebrovascular disease or Lewy body pathology) would be solved and uniformity of definitions could assist in constructing trial populations and comparing results across trials [11].

However, the new definition needs to be compared with the traditional dual neuropathological diagnosis before establishing its validity as a new gold standard.

References

[1]   Bouwman FH, Verwey NA, Klein M et al. New research criteria for the diagnosis of Alzheimer's disease applied in Memory Clinic Population. *Dement Geriatr Cogn Disord* 2010; 30:1-7.

[2]   Jack OR, Knopman DS, Jagust WJ, Shaw LM et al. Hypothetical model of dynamic biomarkers of the Alzheimer's pathological cascade. *Lancet Neurol* 2010; 9(1):119-28.

[3]   Morris JC, Price AL. Pathologic correlates of non-demented aging, mild cognitive impairment and early-stage Alzheimer's disease. *J Mol Neurosci* 2001;17:101-18.

[4]   Korf ES, Wahlund LO, Visser PJ, Scheltens P. Medial temporal lobe atrophy on MRI predicts dementia in patients with mild cognitive impairment. *Neurology* 2004;63:94-100.

[5]   Bennet DA, Schneider JA, Arvanitakis Z et al. Neuropathology of older persons without cognitive impairment from two community based studies. *Neurology* 2006;66:1837-44.

[6]   Knopman DS, Parisi JE, Salviati A et al. Neuropathology of cognitively normal elderly. *J Neuropathol Exp Neurol* 2003;62:1087-95.

[7] Dubois B, Feldman HH, Jacova C et al. Research criteria for the diagnosis of Alzheimer's disease: revising the NINCDS-ADRDA criteria. *Lancet Neurol* 2007;74:42-49.

[8] McKhann G, Drachman D, Folstein M, Katzman R et al. Clinical diagnosis of Alzheimer's disease: report of the NINCDS-ADRDA Work Group under the auspices of Department of Health and Human Services Task Force on Alzheimer's Disease. *Neurology* 1984;34:939-44.

[9] Cummings J. Primary progressive aphasia and the growing role of biomarkers in neurological diagnosis. *Ann Neurol* 2008;64:361-64.

[10] Alladi S, Xuereb J, Bak T et al. Focal cortical presentations of Alzheimer's disease. *Brain* 2007;130:2636-45.

[11] Dubois B, Feldman HH, Jacova C, Cummings J et al. Revising the definition of Alzheimer-s disease: a new lexicon. *Lancet Neurol* 2010;9:1118-27.

[12] Welsh-Bohmer KA; JS; GJ. *Handbook of Dementia Illnesses*. Second Edition. Morris JC; Holtzman DM, editors. Taylor & Francis; New York: 2006.

[13] Sarazin M, Berr C, De Rotrou J et al. Amnestic syndrome of the medial temporal type identifies prodromal AD : a longitudinal study. *Neurology* 2007;69:1859-67.

[14] Knopman DS, DeKosky ST, Cummings JL et al. Practice parameter: diagnosis of dementia (an evidence-based review*). Report of the Quality Standards Subcommittee of the American Academy of Neurology* 2001;56(9):1143-53.

[15] National Institute on Aging, Reagan Institute Working Group on Alzheimer's Disease. Consensus recommendations for the post-mortem diagnosis of Alzheimer's disease. *Neurobiol Aging* 1997;18(4 suppl):S1-2.

[16] Aizenstein HJ, Nebes RD, Saxton JA et al. Frequent amyloid deposition without significant cognitive impairment among the elderly. *Arch Neurol* 2008;65:1509-17.

[17] Price JL, Morris JC. Tangles and plaques in non-demented aging and "pre-clinical" Alzheimer's disease. *Ann Neurol* 1999;45:358-68.

[18] Gomez-Isla T et al. Profound loss of layer II entorhinal cortex neurons occurs in very mild Alzheimer's disease. *J Neurosci* 1996;16:4491-4500.

[19] Hardy JS, DJ. The amyloid hypothesis of Alzheimer's disease: progress and problems on the road to therapeutics. *Science* 2002;297:353-6.

[20] Fagan AM, Mintun MA, Mach RH et al. Inverse relation between in vivo amyloid imaging load and cerebrospinal fluid Aβ$_{42}$ in humans. *Ann Neurol* 2006;59:512-19.

[21] Jagust WJ, Landau SM, Shaw LM et al. Relationships between biomarkers in aging and dementia. *Neurology* 2009;73:1193-99.

[22] Buerger K, Ewers M, Pirttila T et al. CSF phosphorylated tau protein correlates with neocortical neurofibrillary pathology in Alzheimer's disease. *Brain* 2006;129:3035-41.

[23] Clark CM, Xie S, Chittams J et al. Cerebrospinal fluid tau and beta-amyloid: how well do these biomarkers reflect autopsy confirmed dementia diagnoses? *Arch Neurol* 2003;60:1696-702.

[24] Ikonomovic MD, Khunk WE, Abrahamson EE et al. Post-mortem correlates of in vivo PiB-PET amyloid imaging in a typical case of Alzheimer's disease. *Brian* 2008;131:1630-45.

[25] Strozyk D, Blennow K, White LR, Launer IJ. CSF Aβ 42 levels correlate with amyloid neuropathology in a population-based autopsy study. *Neurology* 2003;60:652-56.

[26] Blennow K, Hampel H, Weiner M, Zetterberg H. Cerebrospinal fluid and plasma biomarkers in Alzheimer's disease. *Nat Rev Neurol* 2010;6:131-44.

[27] Klunk WE, Engler H, Nordberg A et al. Imaging brain amyloid in Alzheimer's disease with Pittsburgh Compound B. *Ann Neurol* 2004;55:306-19.

[28] Teipel SJ, Ewers m, Wolf S et al. Multi-center variability of MRI-based medial temporal lobe volumetry in Alzheimer's disease. *Psychiatry Res* 2010; 182:244-50.

[29] Hampel H, Burger K, Teipel SJ et al. Core candidate neurochemical and imaging biomarkers of Alzheimer's disease. *Alzheimers Dement* 2008;4:38-48.

[30] Patwardhan MB, McCrory DC, Matchar DB et al. Alzheimer disease: operating characteristics of PET-a meta-analysis. *Radiology* 2004;231:73-80.

[31] Braak h, Braak E, Bohl J, Reintjes R. Age, neurofibrillary changes, Aβ-amyloid and the onset of Alzheimer's disease. Neurosci Lett 1996;210:87-90.

[32] Mosconi L, Mistur R, Switalski R et al. Declining brain glucose metabolism in normal individuals with a maternal history of Alzheimer's disease. *Neurology* 2009;72:513-20.

[33] Reiman EM, Chen K, Alexander GE, et al. Correlations between apolipoprotein E ε4 gene dose and brain-imaging measurements of regional hypometabolism. *Proc Natl Acad Sci USA 2005*;102:8299-302.

[34] Ronald and Nancy Reagan Research Institute of the Alzheimer's Association and the National Institute on Aging Working Group. Consensus report on the working group on molecular and biochemical markers of Alzheimer's disease. *Neurobiol Aging* 1998;19(2):109-16

[35] Craig-Schapiro R, Fagan AM, Holtzman DM. Biomarkers of Alzheimer's disease. *Neurobiol Dis* 2009;35(2):128-40.

[36] Tapiola T, Alafuzoff I, Herukka SK et al. Cerebrospinal fluid β-amyloid 42 and tau proteins as biomarkers of Alzheimer's-type pathologic changes in the brain. *Arch Neurol* 2009;66(3):382-9.

[37] Vandermeeren M et al. Detection of tau proteins in normal and Alzheimer's disease cerebrospinal fluid with a sensitive sandwich enzyme-linked immunosorbant assay. *J Neurochem* 1993;61:1828-34.

[38] De Meyer G, Shapiro F, Vanderstichele H et al. Diagnosis-independent Alzheimer Disease Biomarker Signature in cognitively normal elderly people. *Arch Neurol* 2010;67(8):949-56.

[39] Rabinovici GD, Jagust WJ, Furst AJ, et al. Abeta amyloid and glucose metabolism in three variants of primary progressive aphasia. *Ann Neurol* 2008; 64:338-401.

[40] De Souza LC, Lamari F, Belliard S et al. Cerebrospinal fluid biomarkers in the differential diagnosis of Alzheimer's disease from other cortical dementias. *J Neurol Neurosurg Psychiatry* 2010. Aug 27. [Epub ahead of print]

[41] Perrin RJ, Fagan AM, Holtzman DM. Multi-modal techniques for diagnosis and prognosis of Alzheimer's disease. *Nature* 2009;461:916-22.

[42] Morris JC, Roe CM, Grant EA et al. Pittsburgh compound B imaging and prediction of progression from cognitive normality to symptomatic Alzheimer disease. *Arch Neurol* 2009;66:1469-75.

[43] Dickerson BC, Sperling RA: Functional abnormalities of the medial temporal lobe memory system in mild cognitive impairment and Alzheimer's disease. Insights from functional MRI studies. *Neuropsychologia* 2008;46:1624-35.

[44] Buckner R et al. Molecular, structural, and functional characterization of Alzheimer's disease: Evidence for a relationship between default activity, amyloid and memory. J Neurosci 2005;25:7709-17.

[45] Chetelat G et al. Mild cognitive impairment-can FDG-PET predict who is rapidly converted to Alzheimer's disease. *Neurology* 2003;60:1374-77.

[46] Kadir A, Almkvist O, Wall A, Forsberg A et al. Effect of phenserine treatment on brain functional activity and amyloid in Alzheimer's disease. *Ann Neurol* 2008;63:621-31.

[47] Fox N, Warrington E, Rossor M. Serial magnetic resonance imaging of cerebral atrophy in pre-clinical Alzheimer's disease. Lancet 1999;353:2125.

[48] Nordberg A, Rinne JO, Kadir A, Langstrom B. The use of PET in Alzheimer's disease. Nat Rev Neurol 2010;6:78-87.

[49] Barkhof F, Polvikoski TM, van Straaten EC et al. The significance of medial temporal lobe atrophy: a post-mortem MRI study in the very old. Neurology 2007;69:1521-27.

In: Alzheimer's Diagnosis
Editor: Charles E. Ronson, pp. 61-79

ISBN: 978-1-61209-846-3
©2011 Nova Science Publishers, Inc.

Chapter IV

Mitochondrial Haplogroups Associated with Japanese Alzheimer's Patients

Shigeru Takasaki [*]

Toyo University, Izumino, Gunma, Japan

Abstract

The relations between Japanese Alzheimer's disease (AD) patients and their mitochondrial single nucleotide polymorphism (mtSNP) frequencies at individual mtDNA positions of the entire mitochondrial genome were examined using the radial basis function (RBF) network and the modified method. Japanese AD patients were associated with the haplogroups G2a, B4c1, and N9b1. In addition, to compare mitochondrial haplogroups of the AD patients with those of other classes of Japanese people, the relations between four classes of Japanese people (i.e., Japanese centenarians, Parkinson's disease (PD) patients, type 2 diabetic (T2D) patients, and non-obese young males) and their mtSNPs were also analyzed by the proposed method. The four classes of people were associated with following haplogroups: Japanese centenarians—M7b2,

[*] Corresponding author. Tel: +81-276-82 9024; Fax: +81-276-82 9033.E-mail address: s_takasaki@toyonet.toyo.ac.jp, Toyo University, Izumino 1-1-1, Ouragun Itakuracho, Gunma 374-0193, Japan

D4b2a, and B5b; Japanese PD patients—M7b2, B4e, and B5b; Japanese T2D patients—B5b, M8a1, G, D4, and F1; and Japanese healthy non-obese young males— D4g and D4b1b. The haplogroups of the AD patients are therefore different from those of other four classes of Japanese people. As the analysis method described in this article can predict a person's mtSNP constitution and the probabilities of becoming an AD patient, centenarian, PD patient, or T2D patient, it may be useful in initial diagnosis of various diseases.

Keywords: mtSNPs, mitochondrial haplogroups, Alzheimer's disease, centenarians, Parkinson's disease, type 2 diabetic patients, healthy non-obese young males radial basis function (RBF).

Introduction

Mitochondria are essential cytoplasmic organelles generating cellular energy in the form of adenosine triphosphate by oxidative phosphorylation. Most cells contain hundreds of mitochondria, each of which has several mitochondrial DNA (mtDNA) copies, so each cell contains thousands of mtDNA copies. mtDNA has a very high mutation rate, and when a mutation occurs the cell initially contains a mixture of wild-type and mutant mtDNAs, a situation known as heteroplasmy. If the percentage of mutant mtDNA increases enough that the cell's ATP production falls below the level needed for normal cell function, disease symptoms appear and become progressively worse. A wide variety of diseases—such as Alzheimer's disease (AD), Parkinson's disease (PD), and cancer—are reportedly linked to mitochondrial dysfunction, and it is clear that mitochondrial diseases encompass an extraordinary assemblage of clinical problems [1–3].

Although mtDNA mutations have been reported to be related both to a wide variety of diseases and to aging [4–20], there are few reports regarding the relations between all mtDNA mutations and either disease patients or centenarians. The previous reports have also focused on mutations causing amino acid replacements in mitochondrial proteins and, although mitochondrial functions can of course be affected directly by amino acid replacements, they can also be affected indirectly by mutations in mtDNA control regions. It is therefore important to examine the relations between all mtDNA mutations and disease patients or centenarians.

In the article reported here the relations between Japanese AD patients and their mitochondrial single nucleotide polymorphism (mtSNP) frequencies were analyzed using a method based on radial basis function (RBF) networks [21,22] and a modified method based on RBF network predictions [23]. In addition, the relations between the haplogroups of the AD patients and those of the other four classes of people are also described using the same analysis method. The results described here are quite different from those reported previously [15,16,24,25].

Materials and Methods

mtSNPs for Japanese People

Tanaka et al. (2004) sequenced the complete mitochondrial genomes of 672 Japanese individuals to construct an East Asia mtDNA phylogeny. Using these sequences and other published Asian sequences, they constructed the phylogenetic tree for macrohaplogroups M and N [26]. The following was used in this article. Website: http://mtsnp.tmig.or.jp/mtsnp; mtSNPs used: those in 96 Japanese AD patients, 96 Japanese centenarians, 96 Japanese PD patients, 96 Japanese type 2 diabetic (T2D) patients, and 96 Japanese healthy non-obese young males; tissue: blood; sex: male and female except for healthy non-obese young males; origin: Asian.

RBF-Based Method of mtSNP Classification

The mtSNP classification for AD patients was examined using a radial basis function (RBF) and the modified method. The RBF network is an artificial network used in supervised learning problems such as regression, classification, and time series prediction. In supervised learning a function is inferred from examples (training set) that a teacher supplies. The elements in the training set are paired values of the independent (input) variable and dependent (output) variable.

The RBF network shown in Fig. 1 was learned from the training set as the mtSNPs of the AD patients were regarded as correct and the mtSNPs of other four classes of people (centenarians, PD patients, T2D patients, and healthy non-obese young males) were regarded as incorrect. Similarly, in the mtSNP classification for the centenarians the mtSNPs of the centenarians are regarded as correct and those of the other four classes are regarded as incorrect. The mtSNPs of the PD patients, T2D patients, and healthy non-obese young males were also classified this way.

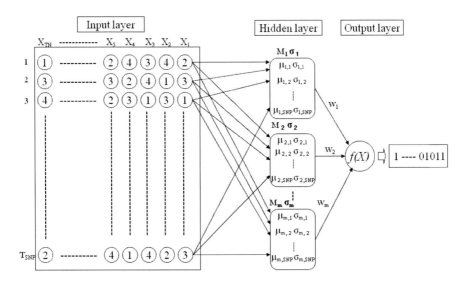

Figure 1. RBF network representation of the relations between individual mtSNPs and the AD patients. The input layer is the set of mtSNP sequences represented numerically (A, G, C, and T are converted to 1, 2, 3, and 4). The hidden layer classifies the input vectors into several clusters depending on the similarities of individual input vectors. The output layer is determined depending on which analysis is carried out. In the case of AD patients, 1 corresponds to AD patients and 0 corresponds to other four classes of people. In the case of centenarians, 1 corresponds to centenarinas and 0 corresponds to other four classes of people. The PD patients, T2D patients, and healthy non-obese young males are also carried out in similar way. X_i : i-th input vector, TN : maximum number of vectors (in this example, TN=320 (64x5)), T_{SNP} : maximum number of mtSNPs (in this example, T_{SNP} =562), M_m: the location vector, m: the number of basis functions, μ: basis function, σ: standard deviation, w_i: i-th weighting variable, $f(X)$: weighted sum function.

The mitochondrial genome sequences of the AD patients were partitioned into two sets: training data comprising the sequences of 64 AD patients, and validation data comprising the sequences of the other 32 AD patients. The training and validation steps are described in detail elsewhere [27].

Modified Classification Method Based on Probabilities Predicted by the RBF Network

Since a RBF network can predict the probabilities that persons with certain mtSNPs belong to certain classes (e.g., AD patients, centenarians, PD patients, T2D patients, or healthy non-obese young males), these predicted probabilities are used to identify mtSNP features. By examining the relations between individual mtSNPs and the persons with high predicted probabilities of belonging to one of these classes, we are able to identify other mtSNPs useful for distinguishing between the members in different classes. A modified classification method based on the probabilities predicted by the RBF network was thus carried out in the following way [23].

1) Select the analysis target class (i.e., AD patients, centenarians, PD patients, T2D patients, or healthy non-obese young males).
2) Rank individuals according to their predicted probabilities of belonging to the target class.
3) Either select individuals whose probabilities are greater than a certain value or select the desired number of individuals from the top, and set them as a modified cluster.

Results and Discussion

Associations between Asian/Japanese Haplogroups and mtSNPs of the AD Patients

The mtSNP classifications for the AD patients were executed by the above described method. As a result, mtSNP clusters obtained were listed in Table 1. The average predicted probabilities of these clusters for becoming the AD patients were respectively 62.1%, 59.4%, 35.1%, 28.6%, 24%, 10.5% and 0%. Then individuals whose probabilities were greater than 70% for the AD patients were selected using the modified classification method. mtSNPs of the 21 AD patients selected were examined at individual mtDNA positions. After that, the relations between Asian/Japanese haplogroups and mtSNPs for the AD patients were examined [26,28,29]. The associations between the haplogroups and mtSNPs for the AD patients are shown in Fig. 2 A. The features of associations for the AD patients were L3-M-G2a (38%), L3-N-B4c1 (19%), and N9b1 (19%).

Table 1. mtSNP classifications for the AD patients

	Classification ID	Number of persons	Predicted probability (%)
	1	29	62.1
	2	32	59.4
	3	37	35.1
	4	21	28.6
AD patients	5	25	24
	6	19	10.5
	7	50	0
	8	49	0
	9	58	0

To compare the mitochondrial haplogroups of the AD patients with those of other classes of Japanese people, the relations between four classes of Japanese people (i.e., Japanese centenarians, Parkinson's disease (PD) patients, type 2 diabetic (T2D) patients, and non-obese young males) and their mtSNPs were also examined using the same modified method. The associations between the haplogroups and mtSNPs for four classes of people are shown in Fig.2 B to E. The four classes of people were associated with following haplogroups: Japanese centenarians— L3-M-M7b2 (40%), L3-M-D-D4b2a (27%), and L3-N-B5b (20%); the PD patients—L3-M-M7b2 (50%), L3-N-B4e (20%), and B5b (20%); the T2D patients—L3-M-D-D4 (10%), L3-M-M8a1 (10%), G (10%), L3-N-B5b (30%), and F1 (10%); and the healthy non-obese young males—L3-M-D-D4g (38%), and D4b1b (38%).

The relations among the haplogroups for these five classes of people are listed in Table 2. The common, sub-common, and non-common haplogroups among individual classes are as follows: Common: M7b2—centenarians and PD patients; B5b—centenarians, PD patients, and T2D patients. Sub-common: D4b2a, D4, D4g, and D4b1b—centenarians, T2D patients and healthy non-obese young males; B4c1 and B4e—AD patients and PD patients; G2a and G—AD patients and T2D patients. Non-common: N9b1—AD patients; M8a1 and F1 – T2D patients. In the case of the mtSNP analysis for greater than 70% predicted persons, as a whole, there were a few common haplogroups among the five classes of people. The centenarians have the common haplogroups M7b2 and B5b with the PD patients and haplogroup B5b with T2D patients.

On the other hand, AD patients do not have the common haplogroups with other four classes of people.

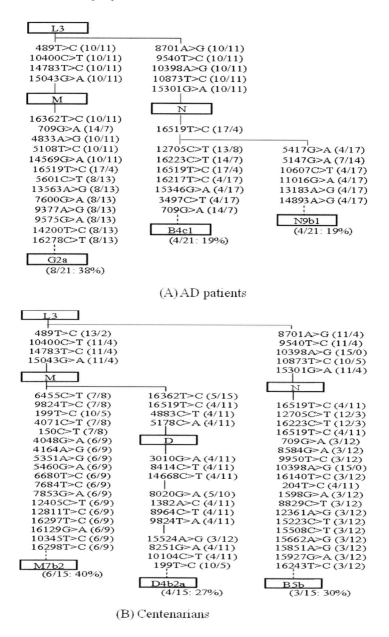

(A) AD patients

(B) Centenarians

Figure 2. (continued).

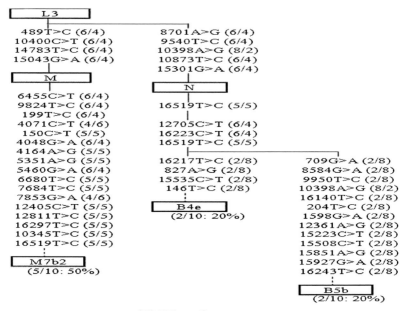

(C) PD patients

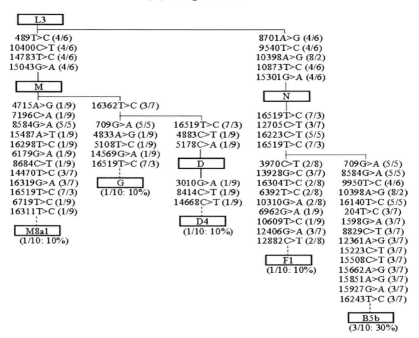

(D) T2D patients

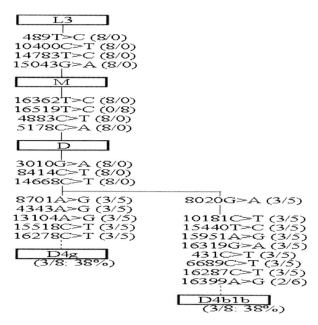

(E) Healthy non-obese young males

Figure 2. Associations between Asian/Japanese haplogroups and mtSNPs of persons whose probabilities are greater than 70%. Associations between Asian/Japanese haplogroups and mtSNPs are described based on the phylogenetic tree for macrohaplogroups M and N described in Tanaka et al. (2004) [26]. The locus of mtDNA polymorphism (*mmm*), normal nucleotide (rCRS) at the position *mmm* (N_N), mtDNA mutation at the same position (N_M), the number of the mtDNA mutations at *mmm* in individual highest clusters (Y), and the number of the normal nucleotides at *mmm* in individual highest clusters (X) are expressed as $mmmN_N>N_M(Y/X)$. For example, 16362 T>C (10/11) indicates "16362" - the locus of mtDNA, "T" - the normal nucleotide at the position 16362, "C" - the mtDNA mutation at the same position, "10" - the number of the mtDNA mutations, and "11" - the number of the normal nucleotides at the same position. (**A**) Japanese AD patients, (**B**) Japanese centenarians, (**C**) Japanese PD patients, (**D**) Japanese T2D patients, and (**E**) Japanese healthy non-obese young males.

Then the 10 individuals with the highest probabilities of becoming AD patients were selected using the modified classification method, and the relations between Asian/Japanese haplogroups and the mtSNPs for the AD patients were also examined at individual mtDNA positions. The associations between the haplogroups and mtSNPs for the AD patients are shown in Figure 3 A. The features of associations for the 10 AD patients from the top were L3-M-G2a (60%) and N9b1 (40%).

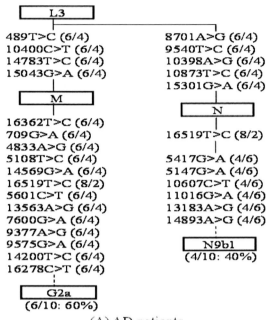

(A) AD patients

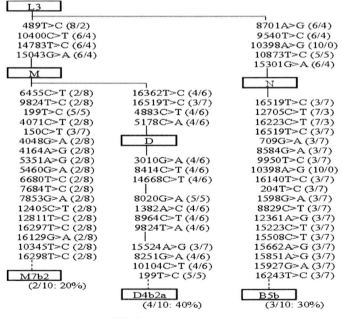

(B) Centenarians

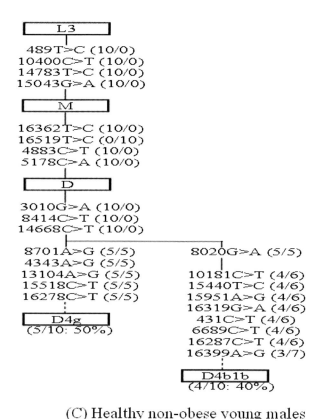

(C) Healthy non-obese young males

Figure 3. Associations between Asian/Japanese haplogroups and mtSNPs of 10 persons from the top. (**A**) Japanese AD patients, (**B**) Japanese centenarians, and (**C**) Japanese healthy non-obese young males.

The other four classes of people were also examined. As the 10 persons from the top for the PD patients and T2D patients were the same as the individuals whose probabilities are greater than 70%, distributions of mtSNPs were only examined for the centenarians and healthy non-obese young males. The associations between the haplogroups and mtSNPs of two classes of people are shown in Fig.3 B and C. The centenarians were associated with L3-M-M7b2 (20%), L3-M-D-D4b2a (40%), and L3-N-B5b (30%); the healthy non-obese young males were associated with L3-M-D-D4g (50%), and D4b1b (40%).

The relations among the haplogroups for the five classes of people are also listed in Table 2. The common, sub-common, and non-common haplogroups among individual classes are as follows: Common: M7b2 – centenarians and

PD patients; B5b – centenarians, PD patients, and T2D patients. Sub-common: D4b2a, D4, D4g, and D4b1b – centenarians, T2D patients and healthy non-obese young males; G2a and G – AD patients and T2D patients. Non-common: N9b1 – AD patients; M8a1 and F1 – T2D patients.

Table 2. The relations among the haplogroups for the five classes of people

Classification consideration	AD patients	Centenarians	PD patients	T2D patients	non-obese males
Persons whose probabilities are greater than 70%				M8a1 (10%)	
		M7b2 (40%)	M7b2 (50%)		
				G (10%)	
	G2a (38%)				
				D4 (10%)	
					D4b1b (38%)
		D4b2a (27%)			
					D4g (38%)
			B4e (20%)		
	B4c1 (19%)				
		B5b (20%)	B5b (20%)	B5b (30%)	
	N9b1 (19%)				
				F1 (10%)	
10 persons from the top				M8a1 (10%)	
		M7b2 (20%)	M7b2 (50%)		
				G (10%)	
	G2a (60%)				
				D4 (10%)	
					D4b1b (40%)
		D4b2a (40%)			
					D4g (50%)
			B4e (20%)		
		B5b (30%)	B5b (20%)	B5b (30%)	
	N9b1 (40%)				
				F1 (10%)	

From Table 2, it is clear that both analyses indicate that the haplogroups of the AD patients are different from those of other four classes of Japanese people. Furthermore, although the haplogroups of the centenarians and T2D patients have been reported [15,16,25], there are few reports for the AD patients [23]. The results are therefore considered as new findings.

Comparison with Previous Works for T2D Patients and Centenarians

Although there is no report regarding the relations between mtSNP haplogroups and AD patients but there were a few studies concerning the relations between mtSNP haplogroups and T2D patients or centenarians, the differences between previous works and the work reported here are discussed based on the mtSNP haplogroups obtained.

Fuku et al. (2007) reported that the mitochondrial haplogroup F in Japanese individuals had a significantly increased risk of type 2 diabetes mellitus (T2DM) (odds ratio 1.53, $P=0.0032$) using hospital based sampling data for large-scale association study [16]. They indicated that there were three mtSNPs in the haplogroup F – 3970C>T, 13928G>C, and 10310G>A. In the present analysis, the risk of T2D patients for the haplogroup F1 was approximately 10% (Fig. 2D). Other haplogroups related to the risk of T2D patients were B5b (30%), M8a1 (10%), D4 (10%) and G (10%) (Fig. 2D and Table 2). There were therefore big differences between the analyses of Fuku et al. (2007) and the results reported here. The significantly increased risk of T2DM was the haplogroup F in Fuku et al. (2007), whereas that of the results obtained was the haplogroup B5b. Although Fuku et al. (2007) indicated that the haplogroup F was the increased risk of T2DM, the F has four sub-haplogroups F1, F2, F3, and F4. In the work reported here, the only haplogroup F1 was obtained by the modified clustering method. The haplogroup F by Fuku et al. (2007) was characterized by three mtSNPs— 3970C>T, 13928G>C, and 10310G>A, whereas the haplogroup F1 by the proposed method was featured by many mtSNPs—3970C>T, 13928G>C, 16304T>C, 6392T>C, 10310G>A, 6962G>A, 10609T>C, 12406G>A, and 12882C>T [26] (Fig. 2D). Furthermore, as Saxena et al. (2006) reported that there was no evidence of association between common mtDNA polymorphism and type 2 diabetes mellitus, the results obtained may indicate new findings for T2D patients [24].

In addition, Alexe et al. (2007) reported the associations between Asian haplogroups and the longevity of Japanese people using the same GiiB data [15]. They showed the enrichment of longevity phenotype in mtDNA haplogroups D4b2b, D4a, and D5 in the Japanese population using statistical techniques (t-test and P-value). However, the results here showed that the haplogroups M7b2, D4b2a, and B5b were associated with Japanese centenarians. There is therefore no common haplogroup in both methods. Alexe et al. (2007) showed that the haplogroup D5 was characterized by mtSNPs 11944T>C, 12026A>G, 1107T>C, 5301A>G, 10397A>G, and 752C>T, whereas there was no frequency in the corresponding mtSNPs in the present analysis. Although they reported that the centenarian enrichment was not found in the haplogroup D4b2a, the present results showed that the corresponding D4b2a was characterized by many mtSNPs with a frequency of 40% (Fig. 3B). Although Alexe et al. (2007) described that there was no haplogroup having mtSNPs significantly enriched in centenarians other than D mega-group in M macrohaplogroup, the present analysis indicated that the haplogroup M7b2 was characterized by many mtSNPs (Fig. 2B and 3B). They also reported that there was no enrichment haplogroup for centenarians in macrohaplogroup N, whereas the haplogroup B5b obtained by the proposed method also had many mtSNPs enriched in centenarians (Figs. 2B and 3B).

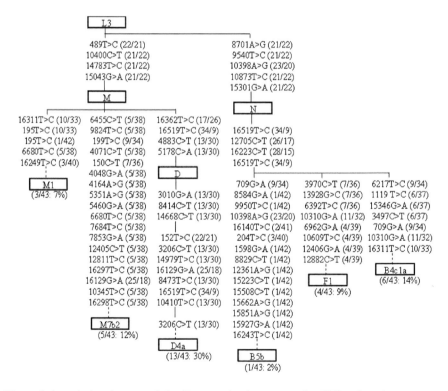

Figure 4. Associations between Asian/Japanese haplogroups and mtSNPs of semi-supercentenarians.

Bilal et al. (2008) reported the haplogroup D4a was a marker for extreme longevity in Japan by analyzing the complete mtDNA sequences from 112

Japanese semi-supercentenarians (aged over 105 years old) combined with previously published data [25]. These semi-supercentenarians were also examined using the proposed method. Since the predicted probabilities of individual clusters for the semi-supercentenarians were lower than those of the centenarians, 43 individuals with predicted probabilities over 46% (the average is 54%) were selected. The obtained results were the haplogroups D4a (30%), B4c1a (14%), M7b2 (12%), F1 (9%), M1 (7%) and B5b (2%) shown in Fig. 4. As the highest haplogroup was D4a, this was the same as the marker described by Bilal et al. (2008) [25]. However, there are other haplogroups indicating the characteristics of semi-supercentenarians. This means that other haplogroups also have the possibilities of becoming semi-supercentenarians. The common haplogroups between the centenarians and semi-supercentenarians were M7b2 and B5b.

Differences between Statistical Technique and the Proposed Method

Although the haplogroups of the AD patients were obtained by the modified RBF method, there are clear differences between the previously reported statistical technique and the method described here. As the previously reported methods analyzed the relations between mtSNPs and Japanese AD patients, centenarians, PD patients, T2D patients, or semi-supercentenarians using standard statistical techniques [15,16,25], they could not indicate mutual relations among the other classes of people—centenarians, PD patients, T2D patients and healthy non-obese young males. On the other hand, the proposed method was able to show differences and mutual relations among these classes of people. In addition, the prediction probabilities of associations between mtSNPs and these classes of people cannot be obtained by the statistical techniques used in the previous methods, whereas the method proposed is able to compute them based on learning mtSNPs of individual classes.

It is considered that the relations among individual mtSNPs for these classes of people should be analyzed as mutual mtSNP connections in the entire mtSNPs. A learning method, a RBF network, was therefore adopted for extracting individual characteristics from the entire mtSNPs, although the previous methods used standard statistical techniques.

The differences between standard statistical technique and the proposed method are listed in Table 3. In the statistical technique, odds ratios or relative risks are analyzed based on the relative relations between target and control data at each polymorphic mtDNA locus.

Table 3. Differences between statistical technique the proposed (modified RBF) method

	Statistical technique	Proposed method
Technique	Relative relations between target and normal data	Supervised learning (RBF) by using correct and incorrect data
Analysis position	Each locus of mtDNA polymorphisms (independent position)	Entire loci of mtDNA polymorphisms (succesive positions)
Input (required data)	Target (individual cases) and control (normal data)	Correct (individual cases) and incorrect (others except correct)
Output (results)	Odds ratio or relative risk	Clusters with predictions
Analysis	Check odds ratio or relative risk at each position	Check individuals in clusters based on prediction probabilities

In the modified RBF method, on the other hand, clusters indicating predicted probabilities are examined on the basis of the RBF using correct and incorrect data for the entire polymorphic mtDNA loci. The statistical technique determines characteristics of haplogroups using independent mtDNA polymorphisms that indicate high odds ratios, whereas the proposed method uses the results of entire mutation positions. As there are the differences between both methods, which method is better depends on future research. Furthermore, the method described here may have possibilities for use in the initial diagnosis of various diseases on the basis of the individual predicted probabilities.

Acknowledgments

I thank Dr. Kawamura for his encouragement and technical support.

References

[1]   Wallace, D.C. (1999) Mitochondrial diseases in man and mouse. *Science* 283: 1482–1488.

[2]   Vila, M., and Przedborski, S. (2003) Targeting programmed cell death neurodegenerative diseases. *Nat. Rev. Neurosci.* 4: 1–11.

[3]   Taylor, R.W., and Turnbull, D.M. (2005) Mitochondrial DNA mutations in human disease. *Nat. Rev. Genet.* 6: 389–402.

[4]   Lin, F., Lin, R., Wisniewski, H.M., Hwang, Y., Grundke-Iqbal, I., Healy-Louie, G., and Iqbal, K. (1992) Detection of point mutations in codon 331 of mitochondrial NADH dehydrogenase subunit 2 in Alzheimer's brains. *Biochem. Biophys. Res. Commun.* 182: 238–246.

[5]   Schoffner, J.M., Brown, M.D., Torroni, A., Lott, M.T., Cabell, M.F., Miorra, S.S., Beal, M.F., Yang, C.C., Gearing, M., Salvo, R., Watts, R.L., Juncos, J.L., Hansen, L.A., Crain, B.J., Fayad, M., Reckord, C.L., and Wallace, D.C. (1993) Mitochondrial DNA variants observed in Alzheimer disease and Parkinson disease patients. *Genomics* 17: 171–184.

[6]   Kosel, S., Egensperger, R., Mehraein, P., and Graeber, M.B. (1994) No association of mutations at nucleotide 5460 of mitochondrial NADH dehydrogenase with Alzheimer's disease. *Biochem. Biophys. Res. Commun.* 203: 745–749.

[7]   Mayr-Wohlfart, U., Paulus, C., and Rodel, G. (1996) Mitochondrial DNA mutations in multiple sclerosis patients with severe optic involvement. *Acta. Neurol. Scand.* 94: 167–171.

[8]   Schnopp, N.M., Kosel, S., Egensperger, R., and Graeber, M.B. (1996) Regional heterogeneity of mtDNA hetroplasmy in parkinsonian brain. *Clin. Neuropathol.* 15: 348–352.

[9]   Simon, D.K., Mayeux, R., Marder, K., Kowall, N.W., Beal, M.F., and Jons, D.R. (2000) Mitochondrial DNA mutations in complex I and tRNA genes in Parkinson's disease. *Neurology* 54: 703–709.

[10] Tanaka, M., Fuku, N., Takeyasu, T Guo, L.J., Hirose, R., Kurata, M., Borgeld, H.J., Yamada, Y., Maruyama, W., Arai, Y., Hirose, N., Oshida, Y., Sato, Y., Hattori, N., Mizuno, Y., Iwata, S., and Yagi, K. (2002) Golden mean to longevity: rareness of mitochondrial cytochrome b variants in centenarians but not in patients with Parkinson's disease. *J. Neurosci. Res.* 70: 347–355.

[11] Dawson, T.M., and Dawson, V.L. (2003) Molecular pathway of neurodegeneration in Parkinson's disease. *Science* 302: 819–822.

[12] Ross, O.A., MaCormack, R., Maxwell, L.D., Duguid, R.A., Quinn, D.J., Barnett, Y.A., Rea, I.M., El-Agnaf, O.M., Gibson, J.M., Wallace, A., Middleton, D., and Curran, M.D. (2003) mt4216C variant in linkage with the mtDNA TJ cluster may confer a susceptibility to mitochondrial dysfunction resulting in an increased risk of Parkinson's disease in the Irish. *Exp. Gerontol.* 38: 397–405.

[13] Lustbader, J.W., Cirilli, M., Lin, C., Xu, H.W., Takuma, K., Wang, N., Caspersen, C., Chen, X., Pollak, S., Chaney, M., Trinchese, F., Liu, S., Gunn-Moore, F., Lue, L.F., Walker, D.G., Kuppusamy, P., Zewier, Z.L., Arancio, O., Stern, D., Yan, S.S., and Wu, H. (2004) ABAD directly links Aβ to mitochondrial toxicity in Alzheimer's disease. *Science* 304: 448–452.

[14] Niemi, A.K., Moilanen, J.S., Tanaka M., Hervonen, A., Hurme, M., Lehtimaki, T., Arai, Y., Hirose, N., and Majamaa, K.A. (2005) A combination of three common inherited mitochondrial DNA polymorphisms promotes longevity in Finnish and Japanese subjects. *Eur. J. Hum. Genet.* 13: 166–170.

[15] Alexe, G., Fuku, N., Bilal, E., Ueno, H., Nishigaki, Y., Fujita, Y., Ito, M., Arai, Y., Hirose, N., Bhanot, G., and Tanaka, M. (2007) Enrichment of longevity phenotype in mtDNA haplogroups D4b2b, D4a, and D4 in the Japanese population. *Hum. Genet.* 121: 347–356.

[16] Fuku, N., Park, K.S., Yamada, Y., Nishigaki, Y., Cho, Y.M., Matsuo, H., Segawa, T., Watanabe, S., Kato, K., Yokoi, K., Nozawa, Y., Lee, K.H., and Tanaka, M. (2007) Mitochondrial haplogroup N9a confers resistance against type 2 diabetes in Asians. *Am. J. Hum. Genet.* 80: 407–415.

[17] Chinnery, P.F., Mowbray, C., Patel, S.K., Elson, J.L., Sampson, M., Hitman, G.A., McCarthy, M.I., Hattersley, A.T., and Walker, M. (2008) Mitochondrial DNA haplogroups and type 2 diabetes: a study of 897 cases and 1010 controls. *J. Med. Genet.* 44(6): e80.

[18] Kim, W., Yoo, T.K., Shin, D.J., Rho, H.W., Jin, H.J., Kim, E.T., and Bae, Y.S. (2008) Mitochondrial haplogroup analysis reveals no association between the common genetic lineages and prostate cancer in the Korean population. *PLoS ONE* 3(5): e2211.

[19] Maruszak, A., Canter, J.A., Styczynska, M., Zekanowski, C., and Barcikowska, M. (2008) Mitochondrial haplogroup H and Alzheimer's disease—Is there a connection? *Neurobiol. Aging. doi*: 10.1016.

[20] Feder, J., Blech, I., Ovadia, O., Amar, S., Wainstein, J., Raz, I., Dadon, S., Arking, D.E., Glaser, B., and Mishmar, D. (2008) Differences in mtDNA haplogroup distribution among 3 Jewish populations alter susceptibility to T2DM complications. *BMC Genomics* 9: 198.

[21] Poggio, T., and Girosi, F. (1990) Networks for approximation and learning. *Proc. IEEE* 78: 1481–1497.

[22] Wu. C.H., and McLarty, J.W. (2000) *Neural Networks and Genome Informatics* (Elsevier Science Ltd., NY).

[23] Takasaki S (2009) Mitochondrial haplogroups associated with Japanese centenarians, Alzheimer's patients, Parkinson's patients, type 2 diabetic patients and healthy non-obese young males. *J. Genetics and Genomics.* 36: 425–434.

[24] Saxena, R., de Bakker, P.I., Singer, K., Mootha, V., Burtt, N., Hirschhorn, J.N., Gaudet, D., Isomaa, B., Daly, M.J., Groop, L., Ardlie, K.G., and Altshuler, D. (2006) Comprehensive association testing of common mitochondrial DNA variation in metabolic disease. *Am. J. Hum. Genet.* 79: 54–61.

[25] Bilal, E., Rabadan, R., Alexe, G., Fuku, N., Ueno, H., Nishigaki, Y., Fujita, Y., Ito, M., Arai, Y., Hirose, N., Ruckenstein, A., Bhanot, G., and Tanaka, M. (2008) Mitochondrial DNA haplogroup D4a is a marker for extreme longevity in Japan. *PLoS ONE* 3(6): e2421.

[26] Tanaka, M., Cabrera, V.M., Gonzalez, A.M., Larruga, J.M., Takeyasu, T., Fuku, N., Guo, L.J., Hirose, R., Fujita, Y., Kurata, M., Shinoda, K., Umetsu, K., Yamada, Y., Oshida, Y., Sato, Y., Hattori, N., Mizuno, Y., Arai, Y., Hirose, N., Ohta, S., Ogawa, O., Tanaka, Y., Kawamori, R., Shamoto-Nagai, M., Maruyama, W., Shimokata, H., Suzuki, R., and Shimodaira, H. (2004) Mitochondrial genome variation in Eastern Asia and the peopling of Japan. *Genome Res.* 14: 1832–1850.

[27] Takasaki, S., Kawamura, Y., and Konagaya, A. (2006) Selecting effective siRNA sequences by using radial basis function network and decision tree learning. *BMC Bioinformatics* 7 (Suppl 5): S22.

[28] Herrnstad, C., Elson, J.L., Fahy, E., Preston, G., Turnbull, D.M., Anderson, C., Ghosh, S.S., Olefsky, J.M., Beal, M.F., Davis, R.E., and Howell, N. (2002) Reduced-median-network analysis of complete mitochondrial DNA coding-region sequences for the major African, Asian and European haplogroups. *Am. J. Hum. Genet.* 70: 1152–1171.

[29] Kong, Q.P., Yao, Y.G., Sun, C., Bandelt, H.J., Zhu, C.L., and Zhang, Y.P. (2003) Phylogeny of East Asian mitochondrial DNA lineages inferred from complete sequences. *Am. J. Hum. Genet.* 73: 671–676.

In: Alzheimer's Diagnosis   ISBN: 978-1-61209-846-3
Editor: Charles E. Ronson, pp. 81-93   ©2011 Nova Science Publishers, Inc.

Chapter V

Leading Role and Limits of ^{18}F-FDG-PET Imaging in Early Diagnosis of Alzheimer's Disease

Giorgio Treglia and Ernesto Cason[*]

Nuclear Medicine Unit, Maggiore Hospital,
Bologna, Italy

Abstract

Early detection of Alzheimer's disease (AD) is particularly important to reveal preclinical pathological alterations, to monitor disease progression and to evaluate treatment response.

The study of cerebral glucose metabolism through ^{18}F-fluoro-deoxy-glucose positron emission tomography (FDG-PET) plays a leading role in early detection of AD because the decrease of cerebral glucose metabolism largely precedes the onset of AD symptoms.

This technique demonstrated high sensitivity in early diagnosis of AD allowing a qualitative and quantitative estimate of cerebral glucose metabolism. Furthermore FDG-PET imaging may help discriminate the

[*] Corresponding author: Dr. Giorgio Treglia, Nuclear Medicine Unit, Maggiore Hospital, Bologna, Italy, Address: Largo Nigrisoli 2, zip code: 40133, Bologna (Italy), e-mail: giorgiomednuc@libero.it

subjects who more probably could develop AD in a high-risk population (as patients with mild cognitive impairment).

A limit of FDG-PET is the lack of specificity; in fact the decrease of cerebral glucose metabolism is a common feature of various dementias. Nevertheless AD patients generally show hypometabolism of medial temporal lobes and parieto-temporal posterior cortices in early stage; other cortices are involved in more advanced AD stages.

The combination of FDG-PET with other biomarkers such as genotype, cerebrospinal fluid markers and tracers for amyloid plaque imaging may increase the preclinical diagnostic accuracy and offer promising approaches to assess individual prognosis in AD patients.

Keywords: Positron emission tomography, Alzheimer's disease, dementia, ^{18}F-FDG, neuroimaging.

Commentary

Introduction

Alzheimer's disease (AD) is one of the most common disorders of older age and represents a serious medical and socio-economic problem. The interest of the scientific community for the AD is now increasingly focused on the possibility of early diagnosis to begin treatment before the onset of irreversible neuronal damage. The pathological changes underlying AD as intracellular neurofibrillary tangles and amyloid-β-plaques appear in fact decades before the onset of symptoms. The early detection of AD is therefore particularly important to reveal preclinical pathological alterations, to monitor disease progression and to evaluate treatment response. Clinical measures of cognitive dysfunction currently used to define the presence of dementia are not able to early diagnose AD, especially in the mild stages [1,2].

This diagnostic challenge can be overcome through the use of complementary tools such as sensitive biomarkers, including brain imaging markers. Several functional neuroimaging modalities have shown promising results as tools for early diagnosis of AD, such as positron emission tomography (PET) using a tracer of cerebral glucose metabolism or beta-amyloid ligands [1,2].

The study of cerebral glucose metabolism through ^{18}F-fluoro-deoxy-glucose positron emission tomography (FDG-PET) plays a leading role in early detection of AD, because the decrease of cerebral glucose metabolism largely precedes the onset of symptoms; thus FDG-PET has become an excellent tool for early detection and estimation of increased risk for future dementia [1,2].

The aim of this overview is to describe the recent developments of FDG-PET imaging in early diagnosis of AD.

Brief History and Recent Developments of FDG-PET in AD

Nearly 30 years have passed since the publication of the first scientific paper on the application of FDG-PET in dementia [3] and during this time this technique has been widely used. For the period from the early 1980's to the present, nearly 300 papers published with the keywords 'FDG' and 'Alzheimer' can be retrieved from PubMed/MEDLINE.

In 2001 Silverman et al. demonstrated that in patients presenting with cognitive symptoms of dementia, regional brain metabolism studied with FDG-PET was a sensitive indicator of AD and neurodegenerative disease in general. Among patients with neuropathologically based diagnoses, FDG-PET identified patients with AD and patients with any neurodegenerative disease with a sensitivity of 94% and specificities of 73% and 78%, respectively. A negative FDG-PET scan indicated that pathologic progression of cognitive impairment during the mean 3-year follow-up was unlikely to occur [4].

In mostly small single-center studies, AD is associated with characteristic and progressive reductions in FDG-PET uptake. The Alzheimer's Disease Neuroimaging Initiative (ADNI) project, born in 2003 and involving many investigators, has clearly demonstrated the feasibility and utility of multicentre PET studies in the study of aging and dementia [5].

Neuropathology and structural magnetic resonance imaging (MRI) studies have pointed to the medial temporal lobe as the brain region earliest affected in AD. MRI findings provided strong evidence that in mild cognitive impairments (MCI), AD-related volume losses can be reproducibly detected in the hippocampus, the entorhinal cortex and, to a lesser extent, the parahippocampal gyrus. In 2005 an interesting review underlined that glucose metabolism reductions revealed by FDG-PET in the medial temporal lobe, parietotemporal and posterior cingulate cortices are the hallmarks of AD. FDG-PET showed a 90% overall sensitivity in identifying AD, although specificity in differentiating AD from other dementias was lower [6].

In 2008 a multicenter study examined FDG-PET in the differential diagnosis of AD, frontotemporal dementia (FTD), and dementia with Lewy bodies (DLB) from normal aging and from each other and the relation of disease-specific patterns to MCI. The authors examined FDG-PET scans of 548 subjects, including 110 healthy elderly individuals (NC), 114 MCI, 199 AD, 98 FTD, and 27 DLB patients, collected at seven participating centers. Standardized disease-specific PET patterns were developed and correctly classified 95% AD, 92% DLB, 94% FTD, and 94% NC. MCI patients showed primarily posterior cingulate cortex and hippocampal hypometabolism (81%), whereas neocortical abnormalities varied according to neuropsychological profiles. An AD PET pattern was observed in 79% MCI with deficits in multiple cognitive domains and 31% amnestic MCI. FDG-PET heterogeneity in MCI with nonmemory deficits ranged from absent hypometabolism to FTD and DLB PET patterns. On the basis of these findings the authors demonstrated that standardized automated analysis of FDG-PET scans may provide an objective and sensitive support to the clinical diagnosis in early dementia [7].

In 2009 an interesting study was designed to evaluate the diagnostic accuracy of FDG-PET in the differential diagnosis of early-onset AD and other dementias in a community-dwelling population that may be representative of patients in the general population. A prospective sample of 102 individuals presenting consecutively to a primary care centre for examination of suspected early-onset dementing diseases was evaluated using standard clinical criteria for the diagnosis of dementia. Functional neuroimaging data was obtained and nuclear medicine physicians blind to the clinical diagnosis generated FDG-PET diagnoses. Final clinical diagnoses based on all available data were then established and compared against PET diagnoses. Forty-nine patients received a final clinical diagnosis of early-stage AD; there were 29 non-AD demented patients, 11 depressed patients and a miscellaneous group of 13 patients. Among patients with AD, the sensitivity and specificity of FDG-PET was 78% (95% CI: 66-90%) and 81% (95% CI: 68-86%), respectively. The specificity of FDG-PET in the differential diagnosis of other dementias, including FTD, was greater than 95%, suggesting that this technique might help in the diagnosis of FTD and other forms of early-onset dementia [8].

In the same year Langbaum et al., within the large ADNI, compared baseline FDG uptake measurements from 74 probable AD patients and 142 amnestic MCI patients to those from 82 normal controls, using statistic parametric mapping. In comparison with normal controls, the probable AD and amnestic MCI groups each had significantly lower FDG uptake bilaterally in the posterior cingulate, precuneus, parietotemporal and frontal cortex. These findings from a large multi-site study support those of previous single-site studies, showing a characteristic pattern of baseline FDG uptake reductions in AD and amnestic MCI patients, as well as preferential anterior FDG uptake reductions after the onset of AD dementia [9].

In the same year, Haense et al. investigated the performance of FDG-PET using an automated procedure for discrimination between AD and controls; FDG-PET data were obtained from the ADNI (102 controls and 89 AD patients) and the Network for Standardisation of Dementia Diagnosis – NEST-DD (36 controls and 237 AD patients). AD patients had much higher AD scores compared to controls (p < 0.01), which were significantly related to dementia severity (p < 0.01). Early-onset AD patients had significantly higher AD scores than late-onset AD patients (p < 0.01). This automated procedure yielded a FDG-PET sensitivity and specificity of 83 and 78% in ADNI and 78 and 94% in NEST-DD, respectively; differences between databases were mainly due to different age distributions. On the basis of these findings the authors demonstrated that the automated FDG-PET analysis procedure provides good discrimination power and a most accurate diagnosis for early-onset AD [10].

More recently Yuan et al. used statistical parametric mapping (SPM) to evaluate the feasibility and accuracy of FDG-PET for clinical diagnosis with characteristic hypometabolic regions, and also examined the consistency of cerebral hypometabolism in AD across different centers at group and individual levels. Scan data including 39 AD patients and 52 healthy control subjects derived from three centers were analyzed and comparisons between patient subgroups or individual patients and relevant control population were performed. In the group analysis, the hypometabolic regions of AD patients obtained from different PET centers were similar and consistent. The common hypometabolic cerebral areas were located bilaterally in the posterior cingulate and medial parietal cortex, temporo-parietal cortex, prefrontal cortex, and the middle and inferior temporal gyrus (p < 0.001). In the individual analyses, the hypometabolic areas identified (posterior cingulated, medial parietal cortex, temporoparietal cortex and temporal lobe) were found highly consistent with relevant characteristic regions obtained in the group analysis and were selected for diagnostic purposes. Complete typical hypometabolic pattern was observed in 67% and 54% of AD patients in two sets of 3D scans, respectively. Only 27% and 33.3% patients showed full typical pattern in two sets of 2D scans. These results indicate that FDG-PET measures and SPM could provide a valuable reference for clinical diagnosis of AD patients. The potential influence of acquisition mode on the clinical diagnosis of AD was suggested for further evaluation [11].

In 2010, Chen et al. within the ADNI project, described twelve-month declines of FDG uptake in 69 probable AD patients, 154 amnestic MCI patients, and 79 cognitively normal controls (NC) from the ADNI using statistical parametric mapping (SPM). These authors introduced the use of an empirically pre-defined statistical region-of-interest (sROI) to characterize declines of FDG uptake with optimal power and freedom from multiple comparisons, and they estimated the number of patients needed to characterize AD-slowing treatment effects in multi-center randomized clinical trials. The AD and MCI groups each had significant twelve-month declines of FDG uptake bilaterally in posterior cingulate, medial and lateral parietal, medial and lateral temporal, frontal and occipital cortex, which were significantly greater than those in the NC group and correlated with measures of clinical decline [12].

Considering that most FDG-PET studies in dementia use clinical diagnosis as gold standard and that clinical diagnosis is approximately 80% sensitive or accurate, a recent study reviewed the evidence-based data on the diagnostic accuracy of brain FDG-PET in dementia when cerebral autopsy is used as gold standard. The authors searched the PubMed/MEDLINE database for dementia-related articles that correlate histopathological diagnosis at autopsy with FDG-PET imaging and found 47 articles among which there were only 5 studies of 20 patients or more. The authors found that sensitivity and specificity of FDG-PET for AD are good, but more studies using histopathological diagnosis at autopsy as gold standard are needed in order to evaluate what FDG-PET truly adds to premortem diagnostic accuracy in dementia [13].

FDG-PET in Patients at High Risk to Develop AD

Brain FDG uptake declines have been observed before the onset of AD symptoms highlighting the importance of FDG-PET as a valuable tool for early detection and estimation of increased risk for future dementia. Thus, the interest of the scientific community has focused on high-risk populations who are more likely to develop AD as compared to low risk subjects. Individuals at risk of developing dementia include: pre-symptomatic subjects carrying mutations responsible for early-onset familial AD; patients with mild cognitive impairment, often a prodrome to late-onset sporadic AD; non-demented carriers of the apolipoprotein E epsilon 4 allele (ApoE-E4), a strong genetic risk factor for late onset AD; cognitively normal subjects with a family history of AD; subjects with subjective memory complaints; and the normal elderly. Overall, the high-risk groups show brain FDG uptake reductions intermediate between controls and AD patients, years before the clinical decline [1,2,14-26].

FDG-PET and Other Biomarkers in AD and MCI

Different biomarkers for AD may potentially be complementary in diagnosis and prognosis of AD. FDG-PET can be used in combination with other biomarkers and this has further enhanced its diagnostic accuracy in AD and MCI [1].

Recently Walhovd et al. combined MRI, FDG-PET, and cerebrospinal fluid (CSF) biomarkers in the diagnostic classification and 2-year prognosis of MCI and AD. These authors found that: 1) all biomarkers were sensitive to the diagnostic group; 2) combining MRI morphometry and CSF biomarkers improved diagnostic classification (controls versus AD); MRI morphometry and FDG-PET were largely overlapping in value for discrimination. 3) baseline MRI and FDG-PET measures were more predictive of clinical change in MCI than were CSF measures [27].

Petrie et al. studied the relationship between alterations in CSF AD biomarkers and brain FDG uptake in early AD. These authors found that in healthy individuals, higher CSF AD biomarkers concentrations were associated with more severe hypometabolism in several brain regions affected very early in AD; these findings suggest that early CSF AD markers abnormalities may be associated with subtle synaptic changes in brain regions vulnerable to AD. A longitudinal assessment of CSF and FDG-PET biomarkers is needed to determine whether these changes predict cognitive impairment and incipient AD [28].

Landau et al., within the ADNI, studied the prognostic ability of genetic, CSF, neuroimaging, and cognitive measurements obtained in MCI patients to predict the conversion to AD. The authors found that baseline FDG-PET and episodic memory predict conversion to AD, whereas CSF measures and, marginally, FDG-PET predict longitudinal cognitive decline. Complementary information provided by these biomarkers may aid in future selection of patients for clinical trials or identification of patients likely to benefit from a therapeutic intervention [24].

Jagust et al., within the ADNI, studied the relationship between AD and MCI biomarkers (such as FDG-PET, beta-amyloid ligand PET and CSF measures) and disease severity. The authors found that different biomarkers for AD provide complementary informations. Beta-amyloid ligand PET and CSF biomarkers agree each other but are not related to cognitive impairment. FDG-PET is modestly related to other biomarkers but is better related to cognitive impairment [29].

Other recent studies compared the diagnostic value of FDG-PET and beta-amyloid ligand PET in the evaluation of patients with AD and MCI compared to normal elderly (NC). Li et al. found that the pattern of regional involvement for FDG-PET and beta-amyloid ligand PET differs in patients with AD, but both techniques show high diagnostic accuracy and 94% case by case agreement. In the classification of NC and MCI, FDG-PET is superior to beta-amyloid ligand PET. Combining the two modalities improves the diagnostic accuracy for MCI [30].

Lowe et al. found a significant discrimination ($p < 0.05$) between controls and AD, non-amnestic MCI and amnestic MCI, non-amnestic MCI and AD, and amnestic MCI and AD by beta-amyloid ligand PET. The paired group comparisons of the global measures demonstrated that beta-amyloid ligand PET versus FDG-PET showed similar significant group separation, with only beta-amyloid ligand PET showing significant separation of non-amnestic MCI and amnestic MCI subjects. In conclusion beta-amyloid ligand PET and FDG-PET have similar diagnostic accuracy in early cognitive impairment. However, significantly better group discrimination in non-amnestic MCI and amnestic MCI subjects by beta-amyloid ligand PET was seen, comparing to FDG-PET, suggesting that early amyloid deposition precedes cerebral metabolic disruption [31].

Forsberg et al. reported a strong correlations between beta-amyloid ligand PET, FDG-PET uptake reductions, levels of CSF biomarkers and episodic memory in patients with MCI and AD. Analysis of the MCI group alone revealed significant correlations between beta-amyloid ligand PET and CSF biomarkers and between CSF biomarkers and episodic memory respectively. A strong correlation was observed in the AD group between FDG uptake reductions and episodic memory as well as a significant correlation between beta-amyloid ligand PET and FDG uptake reductions in some cortical regions. Regional differences over time were evident during disease progression. This study confirmed that amyloid imaging is useful for early diagnosis and evaluation of new therapeutic interventions in AD [32].

Devanand et al. evaluated FDG-PET and beta-amyloid ligand PET in patients with mild AD, MCI, and healthy controls and demonstrated that beta-amyloid ligand PET clearly distinguished diagnostic groups and combined with FDG-PET this effect was stronger. These PET techniques provide complementary informations in strongly distinguishing diagnostic groups in cross-sectional comparisons that need testing in longitudinal studies [33].

About the comparison of morphological and functional data, a recent meta-analysis evaluated and compared the ability of FDG-PET, single-photon emission tomography (SPECT), and structural MRI to predict conversion to AD in patients with MCI; this analysis showed that FDG-PET performs slightly better than SPECT and structural MRI in the prediction of conversion to AD in patients with MCI; similar performance was found between SPECT and MRI [34].

Another very recent study was conducted to reveal the morphological and functional substrates of memory impairment and conversion to AD from the stage of amnestic MCI. The authors found that the discordant topography between brain atrophy (studied by MRI) and hypometabolism (studied by FDG-PET) reported in AD is already present at the amnestic MCI stage. Posterior cingulate-precuneus hypometabolism seemed to be an early sign of memory deficit, whereas hypometabolism in the temporal cortex marked the conversion to AD [35].

Conversely a more recent study of Karow et al. showed no increased sensitivity of FDG-PET compared to MRI in preclinical and mild AD, suggesting that MRI findings may be a more practical clinical method for early detection of AD [36].

Conclusion

FDG-PET, used as a marker of regional neuronal function, has proven to be a highly sensitive method to identify AD and then to predict the development of AD even in mild stages. Furthermore the use of FDG-PET in combination with other biomarkers may further increase its diagnostic accuracy in AD.

References

[1] Lucignani G, Nobili F. FDG-PET for early assessment of Alzheimer's disease: isn't the evidence base large enough? *Eur J Nucl Med Mol Imaging* 2010;37:1604-9.
[2] Berti V, Osorio RS, Mosconi L, Li Y, de Leon MJ. Early detection of Alzheimer 's disease with PET imaging. *Neurodegenerative Dis* 2010;7:131-5.
[3] Alavi A, Reivich M, Ferris S, Christman D, Fowler J, MacGregor R, et al. Regional cerebral glucose metabolism in aging and senile dementia as determined by 18F-deoxyglucose positron emission tomography. *Exp Brain Res* 1982;Suppl 5:187-95.
[4] Silverman DH, Small GW, Chang CY, Lu CS, Kung De Aburto MA, Chen W, et al. Positron emission tomography in evaluation of dementia: regional brain metabolism and long-term outcome. *JAMA* 2001;286:2120-7.
[5] Jagust WJ, Bandy D, Chen K, Foster NL, Landau SM, Mathis CA, et al. Alzheimer's Disease Neuroimaging Initiative. The Alzheimer's Disease Neuroimaging Initiative positron emission tomography core. *Alzheimers Dement* 2010;6:221-9.
[6] Mosconi L. Brain glucose metabolism in the early and specific diagnosis of Alzheimer's disease. FDG-PET studies in MCI and AD. Eur *J Nucl Med Mol Imaging* 2005;32:486-510.
[7] Mosconi L, Tsui WH, Herholz K, Pupi A, Drzezga A, Lucignani G, et al. Multicenter standardized 18F-FDG-PET diagnosis of mild cognitive impairment, Alzheimer's disease, and other dementias. *J Nucl Med* 2008;49:390-8.
[8] Panegyres PK, Rogers JM, McCarthy M, Campbell A, Wu JS. Fluorodeoxyglucose-positron emission tomography in the differential diagnosis of early-onset dementia: a prospective, community-based study. *BMC Neurol* 2009;9:41.
[9] Langbaum JB, Chen K, Lee W, Reschke C, Bandy D, Fleisher AS, et al. Alzheimer's Disease Neuroimaging Initiative. Categorical and correlational analyses of baseline fluorodeoxyglucose positron emission tomography images from the Alzheimer's Disease Neuroimaging Initiative (ADNI). *Neuroimage* 2009;45:1107-16.
[10] Haense C, Herholz K, Jagust WJ, Heiss WD. Performance of FDG-PET for detection of Alzheimer's disease in two independent multicentre

samples (NEST-DD and ADNI*). Dement Geriatr Cogn Disord* 2009;28:259-66.

[11] Yuan X, Shan B, Ma Y, Tian J, Jiang K, Cao Q, et al. Multi-center study on Alzheimer's disease using FDG-PET: group and individual analyses. *J Alzheimers Dis* 2010;19:927-35.

[12] Chen K, Langbaum JB, Fleisher AS, Ayutyanont N, Reschke C, Lee W, et al. Alzheimer's Disease Neuroimaging Initiative. Twelve-month metabolic declines in probable Alzheimer's disease and amnestic mild cognitive impairment assessed using an empirically pre-defined statistical region-of-interest: findings from the Alzheimer's Disease Neuroimaging Initiative. *Neuroimage* 2010;51:654-64.

[13] Durand-Martel P, Tremblay D, Brodeur C, Paquet N. Autopsy as gold standard in FDG-PET studies in dementia. *Can J Neurol Sci* 2010;37:336-42.

[14] Mistur R, Mosconi L, Santi SD, Guzman M, Li Y, Tsui W, et al. Current challenges for the early detection of Alzheimer's disease: brain imaging and CSF studies. *J Clin Neurol* 2009;5:153-66.

[15] Reiman EM, Caselli RJ, Yun LS, Chen K, Bandy D, Minoshima S, et al. Preclinical evidence of Alzheimer's disease in persons homozygous for the epsilon 4 allele for apolipoprotein E. *N Engl J Med* 1996;334:752-8.

[16] Reiman EM, Chen K, Alexander GE, Caselli RJ, Bandy D, Osborne D, et al. Functional brain abnormalities in young adults at genetic risk for late-onset Alzheimer's dementia. *Proc Natl Acad Sci USA* 2004;101:284-9.

[17] Mosconi L, De Santi S, Brys M, Tsui WH, Pirraglia E, Glodzik-Sobanska L, et al. Hypometabolism and altered cerebrospinal fluid markers in normal apolipoprotein E E4 carriers with subjective memory complaints. *Biol Psychiatry* 2008;63:609-18.

[18] Mosconi L, Sorbi S, de Leon MJ, Li Y, Nacmias B, Myoung PS, et al. Hypometabolism exceeds atrophy in presymptomatic early-onset familial Alzheimer's disease. *J Nucl Med* 2006;47:1778-86.

[19] Mosconi L, Brys M, Switalski R, Mistur R, Glodzik L, Pirraglia E, et al. Maternal family history of Alzheimer's disease predisposes to reduced brain glucose metabolism. *Proc Natl Acad Sci USA* 2007;104:19067-72.

[20] Drzezga A, Lautenschlager N, Siebner H, Riemenschneider M, Willoch F, Minoshima S, et al. Cerebral metabolic changes accompanying conversion of mild cognitive impairment into Alzheimer's disease: a PET follow-up study. *Eur J Nucl Med Mol Imaging* 2003;30:1104-13.

[21] Anchisi D, Borroni B, Franceschi M, Kerrouche N, Kalbe E, Beuthien-Beumann B, et al. Heterogeneity of brain glucose metabolism in mild cognitive impairment and clinical progression to Alzheimer disease. *Arch Neurol.* 2005;62:1728-33.

[22] Pagani M, Dessi B, Morbelli S, Brugnolo A, Salmaso D, Piccini A, et al. MCI patients declining and not-declining at mid-term follow-up: FDG-PET findings. *Curr Alzheimer Res* 2010;7:287-94.

[23] Clerici F, Del Sole A, Chiti A, Maggiore L, Lecchi M, Pomati S, et al. Differences in hippocampal metabolism between amnestic and non-amnestic MCI subjects: automated FDG-PET image analysis. *Q J Nucl Med Mol Imaging* 2009;53:646-57.

[24] Landau SM, Harvey D, Madison CM, Reiman EM, Foster NL, Aisen PS, et al. Alzheimer's Disease Neuroimaging Initiative. Comparing predictors of conversion and decline in mild cognitive impairment. *Neurology* 2010;7:230-8.

[25] de Leon MJ, Convit A, Wolf OT, Tarshish CY, DeSanti S, Rusinek H, et al. Prediction of cognitive decline in normal elderly subjects with 2-[(18)F]fluoro-2-deoxy-D-glucose/positron-emission tomography (FDG/PET). *Proc Natl Acad Sci USA 2001*;98:10966-71.

[26] Mosconi L, Mistur R, Switalski R, Tsui WH, Glodzik L, Li Y, et al. FDG-PET changes in brain glucose metabolism from normal cognition to pathologically verified Alzheimer's disease. *Eur J Nucl Med Mol Imaging* 2009;36:811-22.

[27] Walhovd KB, Fjell AM, Brewer J,McEvoy LK, Fennema-Notestine C, Hagler Jr DJ, et al. Alzheimer's Disease Neuroimaging Initiative. Combining MR imaging, positron-emission tomography, and CSF biomarkers in the diagnosis and prognosis of Alzheimer disease. AJNR *Am J Neuroradiol* 2010;31:347-54.

[28] Petrie EC, Cross DJ, Galasko D, Schellenberg GD, Raskind MA, Peskind ER, et al. Preclinical evidence of Alzheimer changes: convergent cerebrospinal fluid biomarker and fluorodeoxyglucose positron emission tomography findings. *Arch Neurol* 2009;66:632-7.

[29] Jagust WJ, Landau SM, Shaw LM, Trojanowski JQ, Koeppe RA, Reiman EM, et al. Alzheimer's Disease Neuroimaging Initiative. Relationships between biomarkers in aging and dementia. *Neurology* 2009;73:1193-9.

[30] Li Y, Rinne JO, Mosconi L, Pirraglia E, Rusinek H, DeSanti S, et al. Regional analysis of FDG and PIB-PET images in normal aging, mild

cognitive impairment, and Alzheimer's disease. *Eur J Nucl Med Mol Imaging* 2008;35:2169-81.

[31] Lowe VJ, Kemp BJ, Jack Jr CR, Senjem M, Weigand S, Shiung M, et al. Comparison of 18F-FDG and PiB PET in cognitive impairment. *J Nucl Med* 2009;50:878-86.

[32] Forsberg A, Almkvist O, Engler H, Wall A, Långström B, Nordberg A. High PIB retention in Alzheimer's disease is an early event with complex relationship with CSF biomarkers and functional parameters. *Curr Alzheimer Res* 2010;7:56-66.

[33] Devanand DP, Mikhno A, Pelton GH, Cuasay K, Pradhaban G, Dileep Kumar JS, et al. Pittsburgh compound B (11C-PIB) and fluorodeoxyglucose (18 F-FDG) PET in patients with Alzheimer disease, mild cognitive impairment, and healthy controls. *J Geriatr Psychiatry Neurol*. 2010;23:185-98.

[34] Yuan Y, Gu ZX, Wei WS. Fluorodeoxyglucose-positron-emission tomography, single-photon emission tomography, and structural MR imaging for prediction of rapid conversion to Alzheimer disease in patients with mild cognitive impairment: a meta-analysis. *AJNR Am J Neuroradiol* 2009;30:404-10.

[35] Morbelli S, Piccardo A, Villavecchia G, Dessi B, Brugnolo A, Piccini A, et al. Mapping brain morphological and functional conversion patterns in amnestic MCI: a voxel-based MRI and FDG-PET study. Eur *J Nucl Med Mol Imaging*. 2010;37:36-45.

[36] Karow DS, McEvoy LK, Fennema-Notestine C, Hagler DJ Jr, Jennings RG, Brewer JB,et al. Alzheimer's Disease Neuroimaging Initiative. Relative capability of MR imaging and FDG-PET to depict changes associated with prodromal and early Alzheimer disease. *Radiology* 2010;256:932-42.

In: Alzheimer's Diagnosis ISBN: 978-1-61209-846-3
Editor: Charles E. Ronson, pp. 95-135 ©2011 Nova Science Publishers, Inc.

Chapter VI

Artificial Neural Networks in Alzheimer's Diagnosis: A Perspective

Patricio García Báez[1], Carmen Paz Suárez Araujo[2]
and José Manuel Martínez García[2]
[1]Universidad de La Laguna
[2]Universidad de Las Palmas de Gran Canaria, Spain

Abstract

A clear tendency of an aging population (2.5 billion elders are estimated on a global scale by the year 2050) has brought about an increase of its associated diseases, one of which is the higher prevalence dementia focusing in *Alzheimer's Disease* (AD). Today, it is estimated that there are 18 million people suffering from AD worldwide, and the disease affects 5% -10% of 65-year old and more than 30% of 85-year old. This situation has important repercussions in the scope of the patient but also in the familiar, social and sanitary spheres. Therefore, early diagnosis of AD is a major public healthcare concern, and the *Differential Diagnosis of Dementia* (DDD) is also one of the crucial points to which clinical medicine faces at every level of attention. The definite diagnosis of AD is only post-mortem. Furthermore, there are not yet a specific set of diagnostic criteria for the confirmation of the diagnosis. In this context it's necessary to develop new alternative methods and instruments of diagnosis, especially on early and differential diagnosis, and introducing its use in all healthcare areas.

This chapter will be dedicated to explore the ability of a complementary approach to face these problems, the Artificial Neural Networks (ANNs). The ANNs are highly non-linear systems. Its more appealing property is its learning capability. Its behaviour emerges from structural changes driven by local learning rules, having the capability of generalisation. In addition to this approach, especially computer-intensive algorithms based on "ensemble learning"-methods that generate many classifiers and aggregate their results are being developed in regard of Mild Cognitive Impairment (MCI), AD and DDD classification.

We will present a study of ANNs, where it will be analysed a new neural architecture, HUMANN-S, which has shown to be a very suitable ANN for Alzheimer's diagnosis scope. The neural network ensemble approach is introduced.

Finally we will discuss the ability of ANN and neural network ensembles, to address this issue, describing the outcomes of implementations of such approaches for AD, DDD and MCI diagnosis using for the inputs several types of data: Electroencephalogram (EEG) type signals, neuroimages, like Single Photon Emission Computerized Tomography (SPECT), and/or scores of different neuropsychological tests, among others.

Introduction

A clear tendency of an aging population (2.5 billion elders are estimated on a global scale by the year 2050 [1]), has brought about an increase of its associated diseases. AD and related pathologies, suppose to be one of the most interesting, not just because of the prevalence of these syndromes (which are estimated to affect between 5% and 10% of people older than 65 years, reaching more than 30% if MCI is considered to be an early stage of dementia in the elderly), but because of the consequences that it exerts on the family in general and on the caregiver in particular. So it is very important to be able to perform early and certain diagnosis and to have well defined all the features related to prognostic factors from the functional point of view as well as from the survival and mortality ones. This way, it could be established the therapeutical steps which best fit. The last end of these actions would be focused onto a better pathology control, and a delay in the functional and behavioral symptomatology, which directly impacts in the patient's quality of life, its personal environment as well as in society.

One of the still open questions in dementia and AD, to which clinical medicine faces, is diagnosis, which precises, to be definitive, the neuropathological confirmation. Using actual diagnosis criteria, it can be considered that ante-mortem diagnosis of probable AD is confirmed around 80% of the cases when this diagnosis has been performed in specialized centers, furthermore there is an important degree of the underdiagnosis, which can reach 95% of the cases in some settings [2], not existing a trustable biological marker for it yet.

Another problematic in the scope of diagnosis and monitoring of these pathologies is the huge spectrum of usual diagnostic criteria, CAMDEX, DSM-IV, CIE-10, and their short coincidence, not much more than 5% in the set, not having specifically validated clinical criteria for each dementia yet. On the other hand, we face the clinical-pathological duality, which according to it can be found brains with a high neuropathological load without the clinical manifestation of the disease. Finally, since a few months, by means of the International Working Group for New Research Criteria for the Diagnosis of AD (IWGNRCDAD) meetings, a new complex terminology has been created [3] because a series of situations, or "diagnostics" appear, even years before the disease starts to symptomatically show, being able to emerge multiple categories, in what to AD relates: AD, prodromic AD, Alzheimer's Dementia, typical AD, atypical AD, mixed AD, Alzheimer's pathology, MCI, AD preclinical stages, at which the presence of a series of physiopathological, topographical or genetic biomarkers are going to play an important role. This described complex situation reveals the need of designing new tools and methods to improve diagnosis of dementia in all their extension, early, differential and of pathology severity level, diagnosis. There has been proposed multiple non-clinicians, statistical and computational methods [4], making a highly interesting scientific field where a wide body of work exists. In general, the ones based on neural computation and machine learning methods are the ones which have supported a great advance in this area. In fact, the suitability of ANNs and the neural network ensembles has been extensively demonstrated for its use in a wide variety of applications where real-time data analysis and information extraction are required, like automated decision making applications or automatic target recognition systems.

We can find a great variety of developed methods, where such variety is framed, essentially, on the following aspects: Types of neural architectures and/or hybrid methods, employed data, different pre-processing used, different number of class of diagnostic criteria (only one criteria class or a heterogeneous set of them), and finally, type of diagnosis to solve. The majority of developed researches are centered in the establishment of binary or bi-modal diagnosis systems, that is to say, they detect the existence or not of a dementia, usually AD, or they perform a differential diagnosis between two types of dementia, usually AD and Vascular Dementia (VD), some front-temporal. Finally, to comment that the neural architectures used are essentially supervised neural architectures and Supported Vector Machine (SVM) based methods.

An important quantity of the proposed methods uses just one type of diagnostic criteria as data, not heterogeneity, and usually just quantitative. The most used ones are EEG signals [5][6][7][8][9]. Other very used kind of data and diagnostic criteria is neuroimage, among them SPECT, Positron Emission Tomography (PET) and Magnetic Resonance Image (MRI) [10][11] [12][13][14][15]. Using neuroimage criteria it also can be found some prospective study trying to develop an automated quantitative tool for the diagnosis of prodromal AD in MCI patients, using SPECT images alone or even combined with FCSRT scores for verbal episodic memory [11]. There also exist researches which make use of neuropsychological tests [16][17][18], but essentially for labelling the data to be used, and other kind of data like form infrared spectroscopy techniques [19], or plasma samples [20]. In addition to these methods, especially computer-intensive algorithms based on "ensemble learning"-methods that generate many classifiers and aggregate their results, working together with data fusion, are being also developed in the last years in regard of CI and AD [21][22][23][24][25][26][27].

This chapter will be dedicated to explore the ability of a complementary approach to face the problematic situation related to diagnosis of AD, Artificial Neural Networks. We present a study of ANNs approach and the most used neural architectures where it is also introduced a new neural architecture, HUMANN-S, which has shown to be very suitable ANN for the Alzheimer's diagnosis scope [25][26]. Finally we will discuss the ability of ANN and neural network ensembles, to address this issue, describing the outcomes of implementations of such approaches for AD, DDD and MCI diagnosis using for the inputs several types of data: EEG type signals, SPECT, PET, and/or scores of different neuropsychological tests, among others.

Artificial Neural Networks

Researchers from different and varied fields have studied the neural processing and control of biological systems and have attempted to develop synthetic systems, that is, artificial systems, which possess similar skills [28], as well as formulating theories regarding how computation in biological systems really occurs. The first ANN model is attributed to Warren McCulloch and Walter Pitts and had universal computational abilities, a formal neural network, based on knowledge that was available on nervous system functions [29]. Since then there has been a series of advances that have placed neural computation as a key element in the solution of a great variety of problems in a wide domain of applications and as a capable computational paradigm for the advanced knowledge in the function and structure of the brain as well as its computation style.

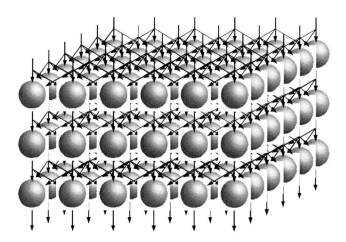

Figure 1. Three dimensional architecture of an artificial neural feed-forward and partially connected network, with one input layer, two hidden layers and one output layer.

Neural computation can be understood as parallel, distributed, and adaptive computing carried out by three dimensional modular architectures organized in layers and made up of a large number of processing elements, with a high degree of connectivity, Figure 1, with a learning ability that may be supervised or not [28]. Its main structure for information processing is artificial neural networks, ANN, where the adjective neural suggests that they are inspired in biological neural networks. ANNs study use some strategies from the methods used by biological neurons to process information. Neural computation is just one of many different computational models that have been defined throughout history, where ANNs are considered as another approach to computational problems [30].

ANNs can be defined as large, parallel and interconnected networks that are made up of simple elements (generally adaptative) and with a hierarchical organization that attempt to interact with the objects of the real world by imitating the biological nervous system [31]. Artificial neural networks found their inspiration in biological neural networks. Thus, there is a biological feel for the models and systems based on ANNs or neural computation. Nevertheless, the task of generating an ANN comparable to the biological neural network is not easy at all, since the human brain has an order of 10^{11} neurons and each one of these receives an average of 10^3 to 10^4 connections, all of which are integrated to obtain a unique output with a complex structure of connections, not completely determined, providing a high and complex processing skill. The type and number of connections that each neuron presents is dependent, among other aspects, on the type of neuron and there are many different types of neurons, for instance by examining their morphology, their cito-architecture, their shape and their functionality. If we compare biological neurons to the logical gates in silicon, they are smaller but need a longer time to generate output, even though there is a lack of slantedness by the high number of neurons that exist as well as the large capability of interconnectivity and working in parallel that these possess. From a computational perspective there is much research to do before obtaining a solid method such as the biological one to implement our neural models. Given that the human brain is much more complex in order of magnitude than any existing ANN, it is impossible to approach this process ability, even with today´s technology.

The general framework of an ANN includes eight components [32]:

- A *set of processing elements* (*units* or *neurons*), each one self-contained, with local memory
- *Activation state* of each processing element
- *Output function* for each processing element
- *Connectivity pattern* between the processing units, where each connection has an associated *synaptic weight*
- Propagation rule, to propagate the activity patterns based on the connections network. It is also called a network function

- Activation rule, to combine the inputs that arrive to a unit with the actual state of the unit and be able to produce a new activation level in it. It is also called the activation function
- *Learning rule*, through which it can modify the connectivity patterns based on experience. It can be based on the development of new synaptic connections, in the loss of connectivity or in the value modification of the synaptic weight values
- *Representation of the environment*. There are two information settings, one local and another global

Following this framework we characterize ANNs in the three following levels: *connectivity topology* (covering the neural structure), *neurodynamics* and *learning*.

Connectivity topology is an essential part of the neural structure of an ANN and indicates the shape in which the different processing elements of a network are interconnected amongst themselves [33]. The structural organization of the processing elements that make the ANN up usually uses layers, taking into account the individual units that constitute it with similar characteristics, Figure 1. There are ANNs with a flat neural structure, with only one layer of processing elements (the input layer is excluded), also called *single-layer* ANNs. In general form, ANNs can have different degree of depth, which is given by the number of layers that makes it up, and they are referred to as *multi-layer* networks. In this last case we can identify:

- The *input layer*, where elements are not usually considered as making up a layer, since they do not carry out any processing, but instead simply distribute the input information to the rest of the processing elements which they connect to. Recall that there are also other neural architectures where the input layer can carry out specified types of processing, tied to the necessary pre-processes the input information can be submitted to.
- The *output layer*, which represents units that provide the output of the network. They can have connections to units from any other layer including itself
- The *hidden layers*, all those that generate connectivity of the network between the input layer and the output layer without direct contact with the environment

The connectivity density of ANNs as well as its direction, where direction is understood to be the information flow direction between two interconnected processing units, namely inter-layers and intra-layers, create a structural taxonomy of the ANNs [34]. Hence we can find networks with total connectivity, where all of the units of the network are connected with each other, *full-connected* networks and the dispersed or partial connectivity, where each neuron is connected to only one set of neurons of the network, called *partial connected*. This full or partial connectivity can also refer to the relations established between connections of the two layers. One particular case of this last category is *one to one* connectivity. Regarding the direction of connections between the layers we have *feed-forward* connected networks, where connections go from the input to the output, *recurrent* networks, where connections go from earlier layers (*backwards*) or other networks where connections tie neighboring units from their own layer, which are called *lateral connections*.

Neurodynamics cover the local information processing that the units carry out. This process is given by the local computation model of the neuron, Figure 2. Mathematically this is expressed with the so-called network function *net* that integrates the inputs $\mathbf{x}$ and the corresponding synaptic weights $\mathbf{w}$ (normally by means of a weighted sum, equation (1), when working with a linear computation model, McCulloch-Pitts model [29], although non-linear models also exist [35]).

$$net_i(\mathbf{x}) = \sum_j w_{ij} x_j \qquad (1)$$

The activation function f_{act} (normally a non-linear function of any type), acting on the function value of the network which allows the dynamics of the activation states of the units and finally an output function f_{out} to be obtained, that are applied to the activation state of the unit provides the output values y_i of the units. It is also possible to store local values inside the processing units, $\Box_i$, that can be used in the calculation of the outputs, which is known as local memory:

$$y_i = f_{out}\left(f_{act}\left(net_i(\mathbf{x}) - \theta_i\right)\right). \qquad (2)$$

The neurodynamics of an ANN can be expressed by means of continuous functions in time or also by using discrete functions. The change of the activation states of the units through time in a network and/or of its outputs can be carried out in a synchronous or asynchronous way between all or some of its parts. One of the most common ways in asynchronous methods is randomize, and consists of randomly selecting the process unit that is going to compute the output. Another very common approach is to follow the topological order imposed by the connectivity, where the computations are performed synchronously from layer to layer, starting with those nearest to the input and ending with the output.

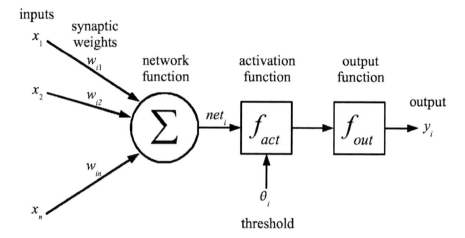

Figure 2. General Building-Block of an Artificial Neuron.

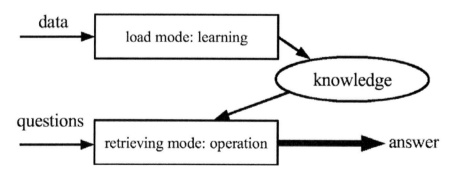

Figure 3. Learning model.

Finally, an essential and differentiating part of ANNs is learning. We can define learning as the ability of a system to absorb information from the environment, without a need for the system to be programmed externally. Learning in ANNs follows a compound model using two stages [36]: *load mode* (learning) and *retrieving mode* (execution), Figure 3. Load mode is where learning takes place. Starting with the data received in the setting ANNs are capable of processing them and storing the extracted information from them, in their synaptic connections. On the other hand, the retrieving mode allows responses to be obtained based on established questions from the setting, by means of adequate processing using the knowledge that has been acquired by the ANNs. Most ANNs models are clearly distinguished by these two stages; nevertheless in other models this distinction is not so clear, maintaining ANNs in a singular permanent learning and operation mode.

Learning processes produce changes in the network in order to try and achieve a new way to respond more efficiently to the specific task. These changes can be gathered by modifications in the connectivity topology and/or by modifications in the synaptic weights **w**:

$$\tau \frac{d\mathbf{w}}{dt} = -\frac{\partial}{\partial \mathbf{w}} R\big(\mathbf{x}(t), \mathbf{d}(t), \mathbf{w}(t)\big), \tag{3}$$

where the function R is called the *instantaneous learning potential* and **d** can or cannot be present, depending on the kind of learning, and is defined as the *teacher signal*, and the synaptic weight vector **w** changes in the direction of decreasing R. We can reformulate and simplify the equation (3) for discrete case as:

$$w_{ij}(t+1) = w_{ij}(t) + \Delta w_{ij}(t). \tag{4}$$

In general terms, ANNs carry out the learning process by itself based on a set of training data sets, which is called learning based on examples, in these cases learning algorithms are used, which are iteratively ordered to update the weighted values and/or necessary topological changes. As opposed to neurodynamics, the performance of non-local processes in the definition of the learning algorithms is allowed. There is also a dependent designer modality, which can establish the needed changes by means of an appropriate formulation to solve the problem.

Regarding the type of learning that can be computed we identify two types of different learning experiences [32]:

- *Associative learning*: where experience learns to produce a pattern of specific activation in a set of units when another specific pattern occurs in another set of units. It allows, consequently, to map arbitrary activation patterns in the input, into other activation patterns into another set of units, normally output
- *Feature detection*: the processing units learn to answer when faced with *interesting patterns* in their input. It is the basis for the development of characteristic detectors and consequently the basis for knowledge representation in ANNs
- Based on the guided learning process we can identify three different paradigms [37]:
- *Supervised learning*: for each input pattern to the network the learning experience is provided from the correct response to the pattern, which serves as a guide for the necessary adjustments in the synaptic weights
- *Reinforcement learning*: it facilitates a scalar evaluation of the response when the network responds to a given input pattern, indicating whether it is correct or incorrect. Many authors consider this paradigm to be part of supervised learning, comparing this to what would be *learning with a tutor*
- *Unsupervised learning*: in this case the network does not receive any tutoring, but has to organize its output based on redundancy and structures that can be detected in the input. This paradigm is also usually called *self-organized learning*

The entire learning process, independent of its type and according to the taxonomy carried out entails a way in which synaptic weights are modified and updated. This way consists of what we call learning rules, which are mathematically expressed, according to the type of systems (continuos or discrete), and by means of differential equations or difference equations. When dealing with the different types of rules we can speak of another classification for learning processes, where we identify four different types [37][38]:

- *Hebbian*: It can be considered as a learning support, biological as well as computational, by constructing the basis of many follow up learning rules, essentially unsupervised ones. It is included in the coincidence learning category [33]. In neurocomputation the Hebbian rule has its origin in the affirmations stated by Donald Hebb in 1949 [39] based on neurobiological observations that indicate that the synaptic connections tend to be reinforced before correlated triggers from the neurons join them

- *Competitive*: this type also has high neurobiological characteristics since its experiments have shown their use in the formation of topographic maps in the brain and in the orientation of cell nerves that are sensitive from the striate cortex. It is based on a competition process among all units to assign the exclusive representation in the face of a group of input patterns

- *Error correction*: it focuses on rules based on error correction attempt to correct the error that is produced in the network when comparing the desired output with the actual output from the network. It is normally applied in the supervised paradigm. The way to correct the error is based, essentially, on gradient descent methods, consisting of the construction of a global error function that tries to minimize movements in the direction of the the maximum tangent. Biological plausibility is not so evident as in the earlier cases, nevertheless this type has obtained very good practical results, and some of the most relevant results from this type are due to the *perceptron rule* [40], the *delta rule* [41] or the *backpropagation algorithm* [42]

- *Energy optimization*: one of the best known of these ones is the *Boltzmann learning* [43], and is featured by the use of an energy function, determined by the states of the individual neurons, which attempt to be optimized. There is a relation with the error correction in the sense that both are based on the minimization of a function, but in this case said function is not defined in terms of the network error. Specifically the Bolzmann learning is considered stochastic learning derived from the theory of information and from thermodynamic principles

Other features of ANNs are their computational skills, depending on the type of problems that a network is able to solve, and another one is their computational complexity, which determines how quickly or how slowly learning will take until arriving at a *convergence* in their results.

ANNs have many architecture properties and functionalities that make them especially appropriate to tackle highly complex problems based on behaviour, non-linear, etc. in real time. Among the most relevant are [37]:

- *Generalization*: ANNs are able carry out a generalization process, based on learning, and solve problems that have never been presented before
- Treatment of Contextual Information
- *Fault Tolerance*: ANNs exhibit elegant degradation, which means that in case of a fault in process elements or connections, the network does not stop functioning, although it is possible that its efficiency is reduced but, as it is the case with the brain when a neuron dies, this does not necessarily imply catastrophic faults. This property is basically supported by the redundancy that can exist between the processing units, combined with the knowledge of the distributed network while searching among the different synaptic connections. Even some neural architecture types are able to take over a rehabilitation process and neural reconfiguration such that the responsibility of the process and/or function of the damaged areas are redistributed between healthy areas, same as it takes place in specified areas of the brain
- *Evidential Response*: responses can be graded, indicating the level of confidence in the network based on its results
- *Uniformity of Analysis and Design*: norms followed in any domain for the analysis and design of applications based on ANNs are the same, which means that uniformity is obtained, which is difficult to reach by other approximations

Aside from these properties we can not exclude the massive and inherent parallelism of ANNs, which allow high speed processing and facilitate hardware implementations, and the propensity towards learning, which is the most important existing paradigm in this regard.

In general, applications which have been most useful to ANNs are characterized by their ability to handle the following tasks [37][38]:

- *Pattern classification*: the data or pattern set that is presented to the ANN is found to be divided in a number of categories or *classes*, and the ANN have to learn to identify the class that a given pattern belongs to from a training set, normally generating *discrimination functions* or *decision boundaries*. This task is usually called *clustering* in the case when no a priori information is available regarding the category that the patterns belong to

- *Function approximation*: starting with a data set, with or without noise, which indicates the input and output of an unknown function, the task tries to optimally estimate said function. This problem is also known in the statistical literature as *regression*. As in the case of pattern classification, when associated classes for each pattern are known, it can be seen as function approximation problem, since both tasks use the term *function mapping*
- *Associative memory*: it refers to stored information that can be retrieved afterwards. The event that triggers the retrieval can be the presentation of a partial or distorted input from the memory content; in these cases it is also called *content addressable memory*. If the input dimensions coincide with those from the output they are called *auto-associations*, as opposed to *hetero-association*, in which the input and output space dimensions are different
- *Prediction*: is based on a time sequence of data that occurred in the past, and predicts the next value in the sequence
- *Control*: process control consists of maintaining a system in operation within a range of parameters that are considered reasonable. An example of one of the most complex systems is the human body, made up of thousands of muscular fibres that must act synchronously, or the brain. Such examples provide strong evidence that solutions based on ANNs for these tasks are compelling research activities
- *Optimization:* it consists of tasks where there are a group of independient variables or parameters and an objective or cost function that depends on these variables, with a series of constraints on the range of the variables. Variables are searched to satisfy the constraints while minimizing or maximizing the objective function. In general there is a multitude of problems in different knowledge areas that can be tackled under this perspective, including the control tasks previously cited, which are clearly related with optimization tasks

Finally we must consider the capabilities of ANNs saturated in its structural organization. Two types of structural organization are generally considered: *monolithic* and *modular.* Monolithic organization, where ANNs are frequently considered as *black boxes,* is often used, and not only with the level of construction of models such as an application level. This structural organization begins to present serious difficulties as the neural networks grow, or when the applications become more complex. In specific cases, the complex problems, efficiency usually decays until a point where it is impossible to solve using monolithic systems.

The term *modular neural network* is used to identify many different types of neural structures, in general it can be even said that any network that is not monolithic is usually considered to be a modular one [44]. Likewise, in the literature we can find other terms that form part, include, or are related to modular neural networks, such as *multiple neural networks, neural ensembles, mixture of experts, hybrid systems* or *multi-sensorial fusion* [45][37].

The main idea underlying neural modular networks is the possibility to solve complex problems in a simpler, more flexible, and faster way. This objective is achieved based on the construction of parts or modules, that would probably be neural networks, and at the same time are simpler and smaller that an equivalent monolithic network. This restructuring allows the task learning to be carried out by each module, usually in a simpler way than the global task and the different training that can be carried out in an independent and parallel way.

We can justify the existence and use of modularity in neural networks from an engineering and biological point of view. Within the field of engineering decomposition in successive layers is fundamental and can be verified independently. On the other hand, we also find that the human brain is made up of different complex structures that cooperate amongst themselves to carry out its tasks, allowing us to conclude that a modular organization in its architecture is present. Thus, we see that making use of modular decomposition to solve problems is not the only area where the field of neural networks can be applied [30].

Simple Perceptron

The Perceptron model [40] reflects the beginnings of machine pattern recognition. It is a feed-forward single-layer architecture with an input layer, which is made up of setting sensors, and an output layer, with the responses sent by the network. Hidden layers are not needed. Its neurodynamics are made up of a network function that uses the classical weight summation for inputs, equation (1), and a step, bipolar or binary, equations (5) and (6), for the activation function, with a transition point which is determined by a threshold value θ_i stored locally in the neuron.

$$y_i = \begin{cases} -1 & \text{if } net_i(\mathbf{x}) < \theta_i \\ 1 & \text{if } net_i(\mathbf{x}) \geq \theta_i \end{cases} \tag{5}$$

$$y_i = \begin{cases} 0 & \text{if } net_i(\mathbf{x}) < \theta_i \\ 1 & \text{if } net_i(\mathbf{x}) \geq \theta_i \end{cases} \tag{6}$$

The learning model that it follows is capable of adapting its weights and thresholds by means of a supervised paradigm using the so-called *perceptron rule*, based on the correction of the produced error in the output layer:

$$\Delta w_{ij} = \alpha (x_i - d_i) x_j, \tag{7}$$

where α is the learning rate and d_i is the desired output.

One of the advantages of this model is that it uses the *Perceptron Convergence Theorem* which guarantees the learning convergence in finite time and that the architecture always allows the solution to be represented. Precisely it is in this ability of representation where the greatest limitation of the model resides, for instance in [46] they discuss its inability to solve non linear separable problems, for example in the case of the exclusive-or problem (XOR).

Backpropagation

One way to overcome the representation limitations mentioned in the Simple Perceptron is through the use of Multi-layer Perceptrons (MLP). A MLP constitutes a topology with one or several hidden layers, and feed-forward connections among its successive layers, either in a total or partial way. In order to represent any boolean function it is necessary that some of the neurons use non linear activation functions (thresholding function or sigmoid function, equation (8)), maintaining the rest of the neurodynamics the same as in the Simple Perceptron.

$$f_{act}\left(net,\theta\right) = \left(1 + e^{-net+\theta}\right)^{-1} \qquad (8)$$

The most popular algorithm for training MLPs is *backpropagation* [42]. It is based on a supervised correction of the squared error generated in the output layer using a gradient descent method. This method forces the used activation functions to be differentiable and monotonic. It begins with the output layer and adjusts the weights of the connections that are affected there, producing a backpropagation of errors of the previous layer to occur which successively corrects the weights until reaching the first hidden layer.

$$\Delta w_{ij} = \alpha \delta_i x_j \qquad (9)$$

$$\delta_i = \begin{cases} f_{act}'\left(net_i,\theta_i\right)\left(d_i - x_i\right) & \text{if } i \in \text{Output} \\ f_{act}'\left(net_i,\theta_i\right)\sum_k \delta_k w_{ki} & \text{otherwise} \end{cases} \qquad (10)$$

Some of the most noteworthy problems are studied in backpropagation, since the gradient descent does not insure reaching the global minimum error, as opposed to the Simple Perceptron [46][47]. Many variations of backpropagation have been proposed to over this obstacle, such as generalization, learning speed and fault tolerance.

Kohonen's Self-Organizing Maps

Self-Organizing Maps (SOMs) [31][48] describe the idea that topographic maps, such as those that exist in the cortex of highly developed animal brains, extract the features of the input space preserving its topology. On one hand they combine characteristics of competitive systems, quantifying the input space in different regions represented by a specific number of output neurons. On the other hand, they maintain a neighborhood relationship between the units of the output space, that is, two neighboring neurons will represent close regions in the input space. Thus these methods will generate a discrete map, possibly with reduced dimensionality that the input space, and will preserve the existing topology in this one. Among the most commonly used methods we find the Kohonen SOMs, although there is a great diversity in their variations. Its single-layer architecture presents an input layer that has a full-connectivity with the output layer by means *excitatory connections* (weights greater than or equal to zero). The output layer is organized in an *m*-dimensional space in agreement with the form that we desire for the map, and the most common is a two dimensional matrix. It simultaneously presents *inhibitory lateral connections* (weights less than or equal to zero) among neural neighbors as well as excitatory self-connections. Said connections are those that facilitate the competitive process while searching for the winning neuron from maximum activation.

Their neurodynamic in practice are usually simplified by carrying out the weighted sum of the inputs and the neuron with the largest value in it, considering it the winning unit, sending it in one of its output while the remaining units would send a zero, equation (11). It is also possible to substitute the weighted sum by euclidean distance, in such a case the winning unit will be that which is closest (higher similarity) to the input vector.

$$y_i = \begin{cases} 1 & \text{if } i = \arg \max_k \{net_k(x)\} \\ 0 & \text{otherwise} \end{cases} \qquad (11)$$

There is unsupervised and competitive training paradigm which follows. The main variations are seen in the modification of the synaptic weights, equation (12), which not only affects the winning neuron but also to a lesser degree the set of neurons in the winners neighborhood N, and consequently being able to generate topological relations. The neighborhood relationship between nodes is normally given by a hexagonal or squared type lattice, whose size decreases during the training period.

$$\Delta w_{ij} = \begin{cases} \alpha(x_i - w_{ij}) & \text{if } i \in N\left(\arg \max_k (net_k(\mathbf{x}))\right) \\ 0 & \text{otherwise} \end{cases} \qquad (12)$$

Also a variant of the SOM architecture able to process missing data [49] can be used. This variant prevents missing values from contributing when coming out or modifying weights. Even so, this way of approaching missing values is insufficient by itself, essentially when the proportion of missing values is excessive.

Their uses range from the projection of multivariate data, density approximation to clustering, having been successfully applied in a multitude of fields [48]. This method acquired the problems previously mentioned of Simple Competitive Learning, added by the fact that a larger number of parameters that can be adjusted are available.

Humann-S

HUMANN-S [25] is a supervised variant of HUMANN (Hierarchical Unsupervised Modular Adaptive Neural Network) [50], a modular neural network that can implement the general approach of the classification process, which has three stages: a) feature extraction, b) template generation, c) discrimination (labeling) [51], in a transparent and efficient way. HUMANN uses a multi-layer neural structure with three modules and with different neurodynamics, connectivity topologies and learning rules, Figure 4.

The first neural module of our HUMANN-S is a Kohonen's s SOM module using euclidean distance. The second module is the Tolerance layer. It is the main module responsible for the robustness of HUMANN against noise. Its topology is a two-dimensional array which has the same dimension as the Kohonen layer and a one to one interconnection scheme with that previous layer. The main objective of this layer is to compare the fitting between the input patterns and the Kohonen detectors. If the goodness of the fit is not enough, the pattern is regarded as an outlier and is discarded. The weights of this layer are responsible for storing the mean (**w**) of the fits between the inputs and the Kohonen detectors when this neuron is the winner. This is a new concept called the *Tolerance margin*, equation (13). The goodness of the representation of a pattern by a detector will be a function of the ratio of the scalar product or euclidean distance between both of them and the Tolerance margin of the detector. The needed learning rule to obtain the weights of the global variance in the degree of the pairing, is based on a differential equation that converges towards said average, to which must be added a decay term to make the final inputs to the system more relevant, in addition to avoiding possible pernicious effects of artefacts or outliers patterns, equation (14).

$$y_i = \begin{cases} 0 & \text{if } x_i \geq \lambda w_i \vee w_i = 0 \\ 1 - \dfrac{x_i}{\lambda w_i} & \text{otherwise} \end{cases} \tag{13}$$

$$\Delta w_i = \begin{cases} \alpha(x_i - w_i) - \beta w_i & \text{if } i = \arg \max_k(x_k) \\ -\beta w_i & \text{otherwise} \end{cases} \tag{14}$$

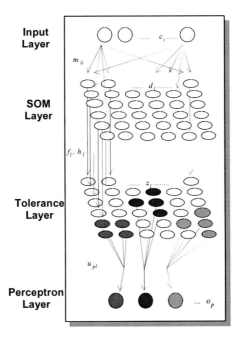

Figure 4. HUMANN-S architecture.

The labeling module is a Simple Perceptron type net and implements the discrimination task. It maps the outputs of a neural assembly belonging to the Tolerance layer, which have been activated by a category, into different clusters represented by labeling units.

HUMANN is available in variants in order to process data with outlier noise and generate not exclusive clusterings, where the input can belong to several clusters at the same time. We can also see the classical Counterpropagation Network (CPN) as a simplified version of HUMANN-S, where there is not Tolerance layer and the Kohonen's s SOM uses the equation (11) as output, and then the Perceptron layer is equivalent to Outstart learning [52]. HUMANN-S is scalable, hence it is adequate to use with large data sets, allowing clusters with arbitrary shapes and those with high tolerances to be found.

Neural Network Ensembles

The ANNs are capable to have several network configurations close to the optimal one, according to the initial conditions of the network and the ones typical of the environment. As each network configuration makes generalization errors on different subsets of the input space, it is possible to argue that the collective decision produced by the complete set, or a *screened* subset, of networks, with an appropriate collective decision strategy, is less likely to be in error than the decision made by any of the individual networks [53]. This has generated the use of groups of neural networks, in a trial to improve the accuracy and the generalization skills of them, referred as an *ensemble, Neural Network Ensemble* (NNE). This name is in analogy with physical theory [53].

A NNE combines a set of neural networks which learn to subdivide the task and thereby solve it more efficiently and elegantly. The main idea is to divide the data space into smaller and easier-to learn partitions, where each ANN learns only one of the simpler partitions. The underlying complex decision boundary can then be approximated by an appropriate combination of different ANNs, Figure 5. The NNE are very appropriate in applications where large volumes of data must be analyzed, in situation of having too little data [23], with data fusion scheme and when it is necessary to tackle complex tasks. Based on the advantages of ensemble methods and increasing complexity of real-world problems, ensemble of learning machines is one of the important problem-solving techniques. The idea of designing ensemble learning systems can be traced back to as early as 1958 [54] and 1979 with Dasarathy and Sheela's paper [55]. Then, and since the early 1990s, algorithms based on similar ideas have been developed in many different but related forms, appearing often in the literature under various other names, such as ensemble systems [23], classifier fusion [56] committees of neural networks [57], mixture of experts, [58][59], boosting and bagging methods [60][61] among others.

Two strategies are needed to build an ensemble system: a) Strategy for generating the ensemble members. This must seek to improve ensemble´s diversity. Some of the two most common methods to maintain the diversity within an ensemble are bagging and boosting, and its successor *AdaBoost* [55][23]. This group of techniques belongs to the sequential training methods of designing NNEs [54]. The bagging method will randomly generate a new training set with an uniform distribution for each network member from the original data set [55]. The boosting approach [60], on the other hand, resamples the data set with a non-uniform distribution for each ensemble member. The whole idea of boosting and bagging is to improve the performance by creating some weak and biased classifiers [62]. When aggregating these classifiers using an average or other mechanisms, the bias of the ensemble is hoped to be less than the bias of an individual classifier.

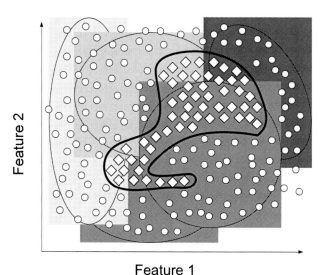

Figure 5. Complex decision boundary from the combination of different ANNs (NNE).

There exist some NNE where the training data is inherently resampled by classifier conditions, as the neural-based learning classifier system, NLCS, [62] or HUMANN based ensembles [63][64]. Each ANN is trained by partial data, which belongs to its local region. There are others ensemble architectures, Stacked Generalization (SG), Mixture of Experts (ME) or GaNEn [27], which also use different designing strategies [55][23]. In this case it must be generated two level of ensemble members; a first ensemble level where individual classifiers are experts in some portion of the feature space; a second level classifiers, which is used for assigning weights for the consecutive combiner, which is usually not a classifier, in the ME, in the GaNEn, and as a meta classifier for final decision in the SG [55]. b) Combination strategy. It is necessary to combine the outputs of individual ANNs that make up the ensemble in such a way that the correct decisions are amplified, and incorrect ones are cancelled out. Two taxonomies can be considered, a) trainable vs. non-trainable combination strategies, b) combination strategies that apply to class labels vs. to class-specific continuous outputs. In trainable combination rules, the parameters of the combiner, *weights*, are determined through a separate training algorithm. In non-trainable rules, the parameters become immediately available as the classifiers are generated. Weighted majority voting is an example of such non-trainable schemes. In the second grouping several choices are available. For combining class labels we have majority voting, weighted majority voting, Behavior Knowledge Space (BKS), and Borda Count Schemes. For combining continuous outputs we can find some other schemes such as, algebraic combiners, decision templates and dempster-shafer based combination [55].

Whereas there is no single ensemble generation algorithm or combination rule that is universally better than others, all of the approaches discussed above have been shown to be effective on a wide range of real world and benchmark datasets, provided that the classifiers can be made as diverse as possible. In the absence of any other prior information, the best ones are usually the simplest and least complicated ones that can learn the underlying data distribution [55]. Such an approach does not guarantee the optimal performance, [65].For a small number of classifiers optimal ensembles can be found exhaustively, but the burden of exponential complexity of such search limits its practical applicability for larger systems [66]. An appropriate design of NNE is where selection and fusion are recurrently applied to a population of best combinations of classifiers rather than the individual best [66].

Methods

In this section we study several methods to dementia diagnose relate problems using three different types of dataset: neuropsychological tests, EEG (ERP recordings) and SPECTs.

NNEs for Diagnose of SLD Using Neuropsychological Tests

In [18] and [27] studies have been proposed new computational intelligent tools to diagnose the SLD of individuals with AD, VD and OD. Using the scores of different neuropsychological tests as input they try to classify each patient consultation in three different classes of SLD. The diagnosis systems are based on ensembles of ANN with capability for processing missing data and data fusion.

Thirty patients participating in a 12-month, controlled consultations from Alzheimer' Association of Gran Canaria. All participants were diagnosed with AD (73.8%), VD (6.7%) or OD (19.5%), due to the data source which does not include patients without dementia. The final and only data set used in this study is made using the results of the 267 consultations. The data structure includes a patient identifier resulting from five neuropsychological tests: The Mini Mental Status Examination (MMSE), [67], is the most spread, employed and quoted standardized instrument to value the cognoscitive function, FAST scale (Functional Assessment Staging), [68], is used to evaluate the possible relation between functional stage and survival Katz's index [69], evaluates the pure function in the basic activities of the daily life, Barthel's index (Bar) [70], is similar to the one of Katz's with the difference of a numerical result, which is adapted for a continuous gradual evaluation, Lawton-Brody's index (L-B) [71] evaluates the behavior aspects of instrumental character. The scores of these scales are strongly collinear, because the different tests are composed of common cognitive components. However, the significance of each test for the SLD diagnosis is different. An important feature of this data set is its homogeneity. Almost every patient has scores from his/her monthly-made tests, with the exception being the MMSE test which is made twice a year. In order to keep the number of tests per year and per patient, the data corresponding to the MMSE have been completed, in agreement with the clinical experts, using interpolation methods. Nevertheless, the data set is incomplete, that is, there are missing data features in many of the consultations as well as the complete patient test battery. Then 74 of the total of 1335 score values have been left empty. The diagnosis of SLD can contain three different values, 15% were diagnosed as Mild, 34% as Moderate and 51% as Severe.

In order to facilitate the convergence, as previous step to their use, the different fields that constitute the successfully obtained information were preprocessed. The neuropsycological tests were standardized between 0 and 10 from the minimum and maximum values that can be reached in these tests.

Those fields not being filled up are labeled as lost values or missing ones, and had a later special treatment.

The availability of such labeled databases is scarce. Then is necessary employ a cross-validation method to improve training and error considerations. The cross-validation variant used is the denominated k-fold, and consisted of partitioning the data set into k subgroups, performing k training exercises, and leaving a validation data subgroup in each one while using the remaining $(k$-1$)$ subgroup as training data. The conducted partition on our queries was based on the identification of the patient involved in the consultation, that is, the consultations performed on the same patients were grouped in the same subgroup. Consequently 30 different subgroups was created, or a 30-fold consultation.

Table 1. Comparison between results for SLD diagnosis for the validation set. (*) both classifiers have 14.98% of errors originated by inputs with missing data

		Best HUMANN-S	Best DTBSE-CPN module	DTBSE-CPN	Best GaNEn-HS module	GaNEn-HS
Sensitivity	Mild	88%	71%	71%	68%	68%
	Moderate	85%	93%	93%	99%	99%
	Severe	97%	72%	99%	72%	100%
Specificity	Mild	82%	85%	85%	100%	100%
	Moderate	90%	89%	86%	89%	87%
	Severe	96%	99%	99%	99%	99%
Error		8.61%	20.97%*	7.49%	19.48%*	5.24%

Two modular neural computing systems employing a multi-net and an ensemble approach were used to approach the problem's of SLD diagnosis. The first system assembles these modules in a competitive way using a Decision Tree based Switching Ensemble (DTBSE) [18]. The CMs for the construction is a CPN architecture. The desired goal is that the system chooses the CPN module that, a priori, offers a more effective diagnosis in that type of consultation, based on available tests to diagnose a patient in a determined consultation. The second system uses a Gating Neural Ensemble (GaNEn) approaches [27]. This system is a new formulation of the NNEs, where the

GMs take part in the combination strategy of the ensemble system, and the CMs for the construction is a HUMANN-S architecture.

The final DTBSE uses 12 CPNs without missing data capability as classifier modules. The chosen classifier modules correspond to those whose results dominate the excluded modules. The final GaNEn uses 20 HUMANN-S. This CMs included in the selection of this group follow the criteria of effectiveness and diversity necessary for NNEs. Table 1 presents the results from the validation of two cited ensembles. Result of DTBSE and GaNEn are included, the best modules of each one of these ensembles (Best DTBSE-CPN module and Best GaNEn-HS module) in addition to the results from the best HUMANN-S with capability to work with missing data (Best HUMANN-S). It is clear that both ensembles obtain improvements in effectiveness that they exceed the best results from their modules. In addition, both improve upon Best HUMANN-S by 1.12% and 3.37%, respectively. These results reveal the effectiveness of our ensembles even when using classifier modules without the ability to process missing data.

NNEs for DDD Using Neuropsychological Tests

In [26] is designed another ANN ensemble systems to DDD. Using the same data set that in the previous section, it tries to distinguish between the two of the most common variations of dementia: the AD and the VD. Then the diagnosis of differential dementia can contain three different values: Alzheimer-type dementia (ALZ), Vascular-type dementia (VAS) and other types of dementia (OTH) that include Trauma, Subcortical, Parkinson and Infectious dementias. The diagnosis systems are also based on ensembles of ANN with capability to process missing data and data fusion.

As in the previous section, neuropsycological tests were standardized between 0 and 10 and k-fold cross-validation was used. Two neural computing systems employing a simple-net and an ensemble approach were used to approach the problem of DDD. The systems are based on classification modules that implement HUMANN-S. The first system is a HUMANN-S-based system and the second one is a HUMANN-S ensemble system, which was combined with simple and weighted majority vote strategies (SMVE / WMVE) [55]. Finally a validation of the systems against the actual diagnosis from a clinical expert was carried out.

Table 2. Comparison between results for DDD for the validation set

		HUMANN-S MMSE+FAST	SMVE	WMVE	Physician
Sensitivity	ALZ	86.8%	96.5%	95.9%	53.3%
	VAS	100%	16.7%	22.2%	16.7%
	OTH	76.9%	84.6%	84.6%	3.9%
Specificity	ALZ	93.4%	89.2%	89.6%	68.2%
	VAS	81.8%	60.0%	66.7%	3.3%
	OTH	64.5%	89.8%	88.0%	9.1%
Error		14.23%	11.24%	11.24%	58.8%

The simple-net designed uses MMSE and FAST test as input. The two HUMANN-S-designed ensembles use five classification modules. They correspond to the following input combinations and errors: MMSE+FAST (14.23%), MMSE+FAST+Bar (16.10%), MMSE+FAST+Bar+L-B (18.35%), MMSE+Bar+L-B (19.48%) and MMSE+FAST+Katz (20.97%). The two obtained systems with this approach presents an error in the validation sets of 11.24%, see Table 2. These results successfully improve, by 2.99% the validation error when compared to the simple-net. Table 2 also shows the values for sensibility and specificity of the best individual classifier and of the ensembles. The validation of the systems against a clinical expert in dementias (Physician) is shown in the last column of Table 2. The final obtained error by the said physician was 58.8%, 47.56% worse than the values produced by the proposed neural ensemble systems. Hence we can observe especially low values in the sensibility and specificity of the clinical expert. These facts reveal the inherent difficulties in the diagnosis of dementias when only using final values from neuropsychological tests, reaffirming the goodness of the proposed systems.

Early Diagnosis of AD Using NNEs with EEG

In [24] seeks the diagnostic identification of AD vs. normal patients based on their ERP (Event related Potential) recordings. The diagnosis of the disease at its earliest possible stages makes the problem particularly challenging. The ensemble approach for data fusion has been used for combining information from different sources, namely different channels of EEG, and different frequency bands.

For this study, 52 subjects were recruited by the Memory Disorders Clinic of University of Pennsylvania. Of this 52 subjects 28 of them where AD patients (μ_{Age} = 79, μ_{MMSE} = 25) and 24 were cognitively normal individuals (μ_{Age}= 76, μ_{MMSE} = 29). ERPs of the EEG were obtained from each subject from 19 electrodes embedded in an elastic cap. The ability of EEG signals to resolve AD specific information is typically masked by changes due to normal aging, coexisting medical illness, and levels of anxiety or drowsiness during measurements. The ERPs of the EEG, obtained through the oddball paradigm protocol, has previously been linked to cognitive functioning, and is believed to be relatively insensitive to above-mentioned parameters. In this protocol, subjects are instructed to respond to an occasionally occurring target (oddball) stimulus, within a series de regular non-target stimuli. The ERPs then show a series of peaks, among which the P300, a positive peak with an approximate latency of 300 ms that occurs only in response to the oddball stimulus, is of particular interest. Changes in the amplitude and latency of the P300 are known to be altered by neurological disorders, including AD, that affects the temporal-parietal regions of the brain [72]. This study suggests that the nearby Electrodes, such as Cz and Fz, may carry complementary information of Pz electrode, the more typically used [73]. Even when the subjects hear, but do not respond, to novel tones. Then three different electrode locations, two stimulus tones, and eight frequency bands were study. Datasets obtained from all 48 three-tuple combinations were analyzed, choosing one electrode, one stimulus tone, and one frequency band.

Before the classifiers training, ERPs must be discretized. Input data provided to the ensemble consists of feature extraction of the ERPs using Wavelet Analysis, by means the Discrete Wavelet Transform (DWT). The DWT analyzes the signal at different frequency bands with different resolutions using a decomposition process. The DWT utilizes two sets of functions, scaling and wavelet functions, each associated with lowpass and highpass filters, respectively. Decomposition of the signal into different frequency bands is accomplished by successive highpass and lowpass filtering of the time domain signal.

The cross-validation variant used is leave-one-out trials, and consisted of partitioning the data set into n subgroups, where n is the number of data values, performing n training exercises, and leaving out a testing data in each one while using the remaining (n-1) subgroup as training data.

In this method, an ensemble of classifiers based data fusion approach is used to combine data from ERPs with different frequency bands of the EEG. A separate ensemble of classifiers are trained with data from each source, and their outputs are combined through a modified weighted majority voting procedure. The procedure used for generating the ensemble of classifiers is the Learn++ algorithm [74]. Learn++ was inspired in part by the AdaBoost algorithm, and borrows many of its algorithmic details. As in AdaBoost, Learn++ also generates an ensemble of classifiers, where each classifier is trained on a strategically updated distribution of the training data. Learn++ specifically targets learning from additional data: it generates an ensemble for each dataset that becomes available, and combines these ensembles to create an ensemble of ensembles, or a meta-ensemble of classifiers.

The five datasets that provided the best individual performances are selected to fuse: NPz_1, NPz_2, TFz, TCz, TPz. All except TFz corresponded to data in the 1-4 Hz range, where the P300 is known to reside, indicating that P300 is indeed influential in AD diagnosis. However, none of the individual data sources provide a particularly stellar performance, except perhaps the Pz electrode with novel sounds at 1-2 Hz range (NPz_1). The individual ensembles were then fused using Learn^{++}, as modified for data fusion applications. There are a total of 26 possible 2-, 3-, 4-, or 5- way fusion for the five datasets mentioned. In Table 3, performance of best individual dataset is given first, followed by the data fusion performance obtained by Learn^{++} combination of individual ensembles. Because of each ensemble had five classifiers (one for each individual electrode), a 2-way combination has a total of 10 classifiers (2 ensembles of five classifiers each one), and a 4-way fusion has 20 classifiers (4 ensembles of five classifiers in this case). Data fusion performance are averages of five independent leave-one-out trials and each trial itself is an average of 52 ten-classifier ensembles (2-way combination) or 52 twenty-classifier ensembles (4-way combination).

Table 3. Comparison between results for ADD for the validation sets

	Best module NPz_1	Ensemble TFz + TCz	Ensemble TCz + TPz	Ensemble NPz_1 + NPz_2	Ensembe NPz_1 + TFz	Ensemble TCz + TFz + NPz_1 + NPz_2
Sensitivity		72.2%	71.4%	63.6%	74.3%	71.1%
Specificit		65.2%	68.3%	89.4%	85.0%	80.8%
Error	25,00%	31.2%	30.0%	24.6%	20.8%	21.2%

Table 3 indicates that the diagnostic performance of the fusion of any 2- or 4- way combinations is better than the performance of the any of the individual data sources. Combinations including NPz_1 performed better than the others, as expected, since the NPz_1 dataset provided the best single performance. Furthermore, NPz_1 and TFz combination provided significantly data fusion performance that the NPz_1 and NPz_2 combination. This indicates that, given the information provided by NPz_1, there is more complementary information in TFz data than in the NPz_2 data. Of a similar way, the 4-way combination of the four best performing datasets did not perform better than the NPz_1 and TFz combination. Moreover, combining data obtained in response to novel and target tones appears to perform better than combining data from target or novel tones only, indicating that target and novel tones may provide complementary information, but only if recorded at different electrodes.

Another interesting observation about sensitivity and specificity is that on average, sensitivity is higher than specificity for ensembles trained with data in response to target tones ($TFZ + TPz$ and $TFz + TCz$), whereas the opposite is true for the ensemble trained with data in response to novel tones (NPz_1 and NPz_2). This indicates that the target tone provides better information in identifying AD patients. This is not surprising, as it is these target tones to which AD patients have difficulty responding. Summarizing the fusion of novel NPz_1 and target TFz data from giving the best overall performance, also provide a more balanced sensitivity and specificity combination.

ANN and Non ANN Based DDD Using Spects

In [75] the AD vs. FTD automatic DDD problem is considered by using functional imaging with SPECTs acquired in different French hospitals. A comparative study between different classifiers, with neural and no neural methods, was performed in order to evaluate their capabilities.

The generalization power of classification methods were checked using 173 brain perfusion SPECT scans obtained from 82 AD and 91 FTD patients. So, it's possible evaluating the impact of the medical centre on the diagnosis of both the classifier and the visual assessment of a physicians group. In relation to the demographic and clinical characteristics of recruited patients, AD patients were significantly older than FTD patients (Student's t-test, $p < 10^{-3}$). Moreover, female proportion was higher in AD, whereas male proportion was higher in FTD (Pearson's chi-square test, p = 0.0025). MMSE scores were comparable between AD and FTD (Student's t-test, p = 0.21).

Images were spatially normalised because of variations of brain volume, shape and position from one patient to another. Determination of a 12-parameter affine transformation (translations, rotations, zooms and shears) followed by a non-linear estimation of deformations required for an optimal registration were achieved using the Statistical Parametric Mapping Software (SPM2). The SPM2 SPECT template used for registration was built by averaging images obtained from 75 healthy subjects (39 females, 36 males). Moreover the data dimension was reduced. This reduction was performed using a brain segmentation composed of 116 anatomical regions of interest (ROI) defined on a single subject brain MRI template of SPM2. These ROIs were manually segmented [76]. After spatial normalisation, the MRI template and all SPECT images were in the same anatomical referential so it was possible to segment all brains similarly. The mean intensity was then calculated for each region and for each volume, yielding a data set composed of 173 patients with 116 variables.

Because of most classification methods require the number of variables to be substantially lower than the number of observations, an additional dimension reduction was performed using the Partial Least Square (PLS) regression [77]. The results were validated also using the leave-one-out cross-validation method.

The Linear Discriminant Analysis (LDA) and the Logistic Regression (LR) classification methods were tested in addition to other four non-linear methods, including:

- *Support Vector Machines* (SVMs) [78]: are a set of related supervised learning methods by constructing an N-dimensional hyperplane or set of hyperplanes that optimally separates the data into different categories. They are closely related to ANNs: a SVM model using a sigmoid kernel function is equivalent to a two layer perceptron.

- Kernel Logistic PLS (KL-PLS): are based on both PLS latent variables construction and learning with kernels. The KL-PLS algorithm can be seen as a supervised dimensionality reduction (complexity control step) followed by a classification based on logistic regression.

- *K-Nearest Neighbourhood* (K-NN-PLS): examines the neighbourhood of an individual datum to determine the group to which it should belong. The data are given to the group that is the most heavily represented among its k-nearest neighbours. This method only need one parameter to be set by the user: the number of neighbours that are taken into consideration (k).

• Multilayer Perceptron (MLP-PLS): explained above, MLP is used with the Early Stopping method as stop criterion that halt the learning when the generalization begins to degrade. Moreover, data given as input to the ANN was reduced by PLS.

All inputs of classification methods except SVM were provided by the PLS components that summarised data variations with respect to the classification goal. Results shown in Table 4 indicate that three methods performed best with the cross-validation: SVM, K-NN-PLS and MLP-PLS. The other methods achieved lower performances. The best classification rate was obtained using the K-NN-PLS classifier with 13 PLS components and 42 neighbours (88% of accuracy).

Performances achieved by SVM, K-NN-PLS and MLP-PLS are very close. Differences in accuracy resulted from the misclassification of a very small number of cases (153 images were correctly classified by K-NN-PLS, 151 by SVM and 150 by MLP-PLS). Comparing the best classifier with two physician's performances (Phy1 and Phy2), results show that K-NN-PLS classifier gets higher performance (the best physician's performance was Phy1 and his accuracy rate was 72%). Therefore, K-NN-PLS method appeared to be more efficient than other classification methods and the visual assessment performed by physician experts.

Table 4. Comparison between results for classifiers and physisicans for the validation sets.

	LDA-PLS	LR-PLS	KL-PLS	MLP-PLS	SVM	K-NN-PLS	Phy1	Phy2
Sensitivity	83%	84%	80%	85%	88%	93%	80%	90%
Specificity	86%	84%	87%	88%	87%	85%	65%	51%
Error	16%	16%	16%	13%	13%	12%	28%	31%

Conclusion

This chapter is a perspective on neural computation approach in the field of dementia diagnosis. The first conclusion we can draw is the suitability of this computational approach for facing this very complex medical problem.

The studies exposed in this chapter contribute advances on intelligent clinical support decision systems to aid in the diagnosis of dementia.

We present a general study of artificial neural networks. This study covers theory and architecture of the several, very used for medical data processing, supervised and unsupervised ANNs. A new modular neural architecture, HUMANN-S, the supervised version of HUMANN, is also reported. We have shown that HUMANN-S is a very suitable ANN for Alzheimer's diagnosis ambit. The NNE has been also analyzed as a successful technique where outputs of a set of separately trained neural networks are combined to form one unified prediction. We have shown it to be a very appropriate approach to the scope of our application domain.

Finally we will discuss the ability of ANNs and neural network ensembles, to address this issue, describing the outcomes of several implementations of such approaches for AD, DDD and diagnosis of severity level of dementia. These computationally intelligent tools are, HUMANN-S based simple diagnosis system, DTBSE, GaNEn system HUMANN-S ensemble systems, Learn++-based ensemble and ANN+NonANN-based diagnosis systems. For each described implementation was used different type of data, concretely, neuropsychological tests, ERP recordings of EEG signals and neuroimage SPECT. Based on the results presented in all them, we can conclude that, the ensemble structure provides a natural mechanism to combine heterogeneous features. Using appropriate pre-processing methods followed by ensemble based data fusion appears to be an effective tool for aiding to effective diagnosis of dementia in all levels: early diagnosis of AD, differential diagnosis of dementia and the severity level of dementia diagnosis. The comparative studies conclude the HUMANN-S ensemble systems provides better performance than the other methods, which means the goodness of this ANN, the value to deal with missing data and the ability of the neuropsychological test, in the Alzheimer' diagnosis scope.

Another important conclusion from this study is the insufficiency of the use of independent diagnostic criteria for diagnosis these type of pathology and the need to use clinical multi-criteria (data fusion schemes) for an effective and reliable diagnosis of dementias. The fusion approach can also be used as a feature selection procedure.

The study presented in this chapter can be an important contribution in the medical diagnosis of neurological disorders, specifically in Alzheimer disease and other kind of dementia. The use of these new intelligent instruments can help to reach earlier and reliable diagnosis , they also can help to alleviate the degree of existing under diagnosis, thanks to its high performance and because it could be used in all healthcare areas, and finally they could help to determine specific criteria for Alzheimer disease and other type of dementias.

Acknowledgments

Authors would like to thank the Canary Islands Government and Science and Innovation Ministry of the Spanish Government for their support under Research Project "SolSubC200801000347" and "TIN2009-1389" respectively.

References

[1]   Tabaton, M. et al. (2010). Artificial Neural Networks Identify the Predictive Values of Risk Factors on the Conversion of Amnestic Mild Cognitive Impairment. *Journal of Alzheimers Disease*, Vol. 19, No. 3, pp. 1035-1040.

[2]   Solomon, P., Murphy, C. (2005). Should we screen for Alzheimer's disease?. *Geriatrics*, Vol. 60, No. 11, pp. 26-31.

[3]   Dubois, B., Feldman, H.H., Jacova, C., Cummings, J.L., Dekosky, S.T., Barberger-Gateau, P. et al. (2010). Revising the definition of Alzheimer's disease: a new lexicon. *Lancet Neurology*, Vol. 9, pp. 1118-1127.

[4]   Foy, C.M.L, Nicholas, H., Hollingworth, P., Boothby, H., Willams, J., Brown, R.G. et al. (2007). Diagnosing Alzheimer's disease-non-clinicians and computerised algorithms together are as accurate as the best clinical practice. *International Journal on Geriatry and Psychiatry*, Vol. 22, pp. 1154-1163.

[5]   Dauwels, J., Vialatte, F., Musha, T., Cichocki, A. (2010). A comporative study of synchrony measures for early diagnosis of Alzheimer's disease based on EEG. *NeuroImage*, Vol. 49, No. 1, pp. 668-693.

[6]   Gawel, M., Zalewska, E., Szmidt-Salkowska, E., Kowalski, J. (2009). The value of quantitative EEG in differential diagnosis of Alzheimer's disease and subcortical vascular dementia. *Journal of the Neurological Science*, Vol. 2833, No. 1-2, pp. 127-133.

[7]   Buscema, M., Rossini, P., Babiloni, C., Grossi, E. (2007). The IFAST model, a novel parallel nonlinear EEG analysis technique, distinguishes MCI and AD's disease patients with high degree of accuracy. *Artificial Intelligence in Medicine*, Vol. 40, No. 2, pp. 127-141.

[8]   Kim, H.T., Kim, B.Y., Park, E.H., Kim, J.W., Hwang, E.W. et al. (2005). Computerized recognition of Alzheimer disease-EEG using genetic algorithms and neural network. *Future Generation Computer Systems*, Vol. 21, No. 7, pp. 1124-1130.

[9]   Petrosian, A.A., Prokhorov, D.V., Lajara-Nanson, W., Schiffer, R.B. (2001). Links Recurrent neural network-based approach for early recognition of Alzheimer's disease in EEG. *Clinical Neurophysiology*, Vol. 112, No. 8, pp. 1378-1387.

[10] Álvarez Illán, I., Górriz, J.M., Ramírez, J., Salas-Gonzalez, D., Lópe, M., Segovia, F., Padilla, P., Puntonet, C.G. (2010). Projecting independent components of SPECT images for computer aided diagnosis of Alzheimer's disease. *Pattern Recognition Letters*, Vol. 31, pp. 1342-1347.

[11] Habert, M.O., Horn, J.F., Sarazin, M., Lotterie, J.A., Puel, M. et al. (2011). Brain perfusion SPECT with an automated quantitative tool can identify prodromal Alzheimer's disease among patientswith mild cognitive impairment. *Neurobiology of Aging*, Vol. 32, pp. 5-23.

[12] Salas-Gonzalez, D., Gorriz, J.M., Ramirez, J., Lopez, M., Illan, I.A. Et al. (2009). Analysiss of SPECT brain images for the diagnosis of Alzheimer's disease using moments and support vector machines. *Neuroscience Letters*, Vol. 461, No. 1, pp. 60-64

[13] Horn, J.F., Habert, M.O., Giron, A., Fertil, B. (2007). Alzheimer's disease and frontotemporal dementia differential automatic diagnosis based on SPECT images, In: *IEEE International Symposium on Biomedical Imaging*, pp. 1336-1339, IEEE Xplore.

[14] Fritzsche, K., Von Wangenheim, A., Dillmann, R., Unterhinninghofen, R. (2006). Automated MRI-based quantification of the cerebral atrophy providing diagnostic information on mild cognitive impairment and alzheimer's disease, In: *Proceedings of the 19th IEEE Symposium on Computer-Based Medical Systems (CBMS 2006)*, pp. 191-196, IEEE Xplore.

[15] Hinrichs, C., Singh, V., Mukherjee, L., Xu, G., Chung, M.K., Johnson, S.C. (2009). Spatially augmented LPboosting for AD classification with evaluations on the ADNI dataset. *NeuroImage*, Vol. 48, pp. 138-149.

[16] Chaves, R., Ramirez, J., Gorriz, J.M., Lopez, M., Salas-Gonzalez,D. Et al. (2009). SVM-based computer-aided diagnosis of the Alzheimer's disease using t-test NMSE feature selection with feature correlation weighting. *Neuroscience Letters*, Vol. 461, No. 3, pp. 293-297.

[17] García Báez, P., Suárez Araujo, C.P., Fernández Viadero, C., Regidor García, J. (2007) Automatic Prognostic Determination and Evolution of Cognitive Decline Using Artificial Neural Networks. *IDEAL 2007. LNCS, vol 4881*, pp: 898-907, Springer, Heidelberg.

[18] García Báez, P., Fernández Viadero, C., Regidor García, J., Suárez Araujo, C.P. (2008). An Ensemble Approach for the Diagnosis of Cognitive Decline with Missing Data, *Hybrid Artificial Intelligence Systems. LNCS, vol. 5271*, pp. 353-360, Springer, Heidelberg.

[19] Griebe, M., Daffertshofer, M., Stroick, M., Syren, M., Ahmad-Nejad, P., Neumaier, M. et al. (2007). Infrared spectroscopy: A new diagnostic tool in Alzheimer disease. *Neuroscience Letters*, Vol. 420, No. 1, pp. 29-33.

[20] Teramoto, R. (2008). Prediction of Alzheimer's diagnosis using semi-supervised distance metric learning with label propagation. *Computational Biology and Chemistry*, Vol. 32, No. 6, pp. 438-441.

[21] Ramirez, J., Gorriz, J.M., Segovia, F., Chaves, R., Salas-Gonzalez, D., Lopez, M., Alvarez, I., Padilla, P. (2010). Computer aided diagnosis system for the Alzheimer's disease based on partial least squares and random forest SPECT image classification. *Neuroscience Letters*, Vol. 472, No. 2, pp. 99-103.

[22] Lehmann, C., Koenig, T., Jelic, V., Prichep, L., John, R.E., Wahlund, L., Dodge, Y., Dierks, T. (2007). Application and comparison of classification algorithms for recognition of Alzheimer's disease in electrical brain activity (EEG). *Journal of Neuroscience Methods*, Vol. 161, No. 2, pp. 342-350.

[23] Polikar, R., Topalis, A., Green, D., Kounios, J., Clark, C.M. (2007). Comparative multiresolution wavelet analysis of ERP spectral bands using an ensemble of classifiers app. for early diagnosis of Alzheimer's disease. *Computers in Biology and Medicine*, Vol. 37, No. 4, pp. 542-558.

[24] Polikar, R., Topalis, A., Green, D., Kounios, J., Clark, C.M. (2008). Ensemble based data fusion for early diagnosis of Alzheimer's disease. *Information Fusion*, Vol. 9, No. 1, pp. 83-95.

[25] García Báez, P., Pérez del Pino, M.A., Fernández Viadero, C., Suárez Araujo, C.P. (2009) Artificial Intelligent Systems Based on Supervised HUMANN for Differential Diagnosis of Cognitive Impairment: Towards a 4P-HCDS. *Bio-Inspired Systems: Computational and Ambient Intelligence*, pp: 981-988.

[26] García Báez, P., Fernandez Viadero, C., Perez del Pino, M.A., Prochazka, A., Suárez Araujo, C.P. (2010). HUMANN-based systems for differential diagnosis of dementia using neuropsychological tests, *Intelligent Engineering Systems (INES), 2010*, pp. 67-72, Las Palmas de G.C.

[27] Suárez Araujo, C.P., García Báez, P., Fernández Viadero, C. (2010). GaNEn: a new gating neural ensemble for automatic assessment of the severity level of dementia using neuropsychological tests, In: *International Conference on Broadband and Biomedical Communications*, pp. on print, IEEE Xplore.

[28] Suárez Araujo, C.P. (1996). Neurociencia y computación neuronal: una perspectiva, In: *Neurociencia y Computación Neuronal*, Suárez Araujo, C.P., Regidor García, J. (Ed.), pp. 251-266, Servicio de publicaciones de la ULPGC, Las Palmas de GC.

[29] McCulloch, W.S., Pitts, W. (1943). A logical calculus of the ideas immanent in nervous activity. *Bulletin of Mathematical Biophysics*, Vol. 5, pp. 115-133.

[30] García Báez, P. (2005). HUMANN: una nueva red neuronal artificial adaptativa, no supervisada, modular y jerárquica: aplicaciones en neurociencia y medioambiente. Doctoral Thesis, Departamento de Informática y Sistemas, Universidad de Las Palmas de Gran Canaria.

[31] Kohonen, T. (1989). *Self-Organization and Associative Memory, 3rd ed*, Springer Series in Information Sciences, Berlin, GE.

[32] Rumelhart, Hinton, G.E., McClelland, J.L. (1986). A general framework for parallel distributed processing, In: *Parallel distributed processing: explorations in the microstructure of cog.*, pp. 45-76, MIT Press, Cambridge, MA.

[33] Hecht Neilsen, R (1990). *Neurocomputing*, Addison-Wesley Publishing, Reading, MA.

[34] Simpson, P.K. (1990). *Artificial Neural Systems. Foundations, paradigms, applications, and impl.*, Pergamon Press, New York, NY.

[35] Suárez Araujo, C.P (1997). Novel Neural Network Models for Computing Homothetic Invariances: An Image Algebra Notation. *Journal of Mathematical Imaging and Vision*, Vol. 7, pp. 69-83.

[36] Judd, J.S. (1990). *Neural Network Design and Complexity of Learning*, MIT Press, Cambridge, MA.

[37] Haykin, S. (1994). *Neural Networks*, Macmillan College Publishing.

[38] Jain, A.K., Mao, J., Mohiuddin, K. (1996). Artificial Neural Networks: A Tutorial. *IEEE Computer*, Vol. 29, No. 3, pp. 31-44.

[39] Hebb, D.O. (1949). *The organization of behavior: A neuropsychological theory*, John Wiley and Sons, New York, NY.

[40] Rosenblatt, F. (1961). *Principles of Neurodynamics*, Spartan Books, Washington, WA.

[41] Widrow, H. (1962). Generalization and information storage in networks of adaline 'neurons', In: *Self-Organizing Systems*, (Ed.), pp. 435-461, Spartan Books, Washington, WA.

[42] Werbos, P.J. (1974) Beyond regression: new tools for prediction and analysis in the behavioral sciences. Doctoral Thesis, Harvard University.

[43] Hinton, G.E., Sejnowski, T.J. (1986). Learning and relearning in Boltzmann machines, In: *Parallel Distributed Processing: Explorations in Microstructure of Cog.*, pp. 282-317, MIT Press, Cambridge, MA.

[44] Rojas, R. (1996). *Neural Networks. A Systematic Introduction*, Springer-Verlag, Berlin, GE.

[45] Gallinari, P. (1995). *Training of Modular Neural Net Systems*, The Handbook of Brain Theory and Neural Networs.

[46] Minsky, M. L., Papert, S. A. (1969). *Perceptrons*, MIT Press, Cambridge, MA.

[47] Minsky, M. L., Seymour, P. (1988). *Perceptrons: an introduction to computational geometry*, MIT Press, Cambridge, MA.

[48] Kohonen, T. (1997). *Self-Organizing Maps, 2nd ed*, Springer Series in Information Sciences, Berlin, GE.

[49] Samad, T., Harp, S.A. (1992). Self-organization with partial data. *Network*, Vol. 3, pp. 205-212.

[50] García Báez, P., Fernández López, P., Suárez Araujo, C. P. (2003). A Parametric Study of HUMANN in Relation to the Noise. Application to the Identification of Compounds of Environmental Interest. *Systems Analysis Modelling and Simulation*, Vol. 43, No. 9, pp. 1213-1228.

[51] Bankman, I.N. (1993). Automated Recognition of Action Potentials in Extracellular Recordings, In: *Rethinking Neural Networks: Quantum Fields and Biological Data*, Pribram, K.H., Eccles, J.C. (Ed.), pp. 69-92, Lawrence Erlbaum Associates, Hillsdale.

[52] Grossberg, S. (1969). Embedding fields: A theory of learning with physiological implications. *Journal of Mathematical Psychology*, Vol. 6, pp. 209-239.

[53] Hansen, L.K., Salamon, P. (1990). Neural Network Ensembles. *IEEE Transactions on Pattern Analysis and Machine Intelligence*, Vol. 12, No. 10, pp. 993-1001.

[54] Liu, Y, Yao, X., Higuchi, T. (2003). Designing Neural Network Ensembles by Minimising Mutual Information, In: *Computational Intelligence in Control*, Mohammadian, M., Sarker, R.A., Yao, X. (Ed.), pp. 1-21, Idea Group Inc., USA & London.

[55] Polikar, R. (2006). Ensemble Based Systems in Decision Making. *IEEE Circuits and Systems Magazine*, Vol. 6, No. 3, pp. 21-45.

[56] Kuncheva, L.I., Bezdek, J.C., Duin, R. (2001). Decision templates for multiple classifier fusion: An experimental comparison. *Pattern Recognition*, Vol. 34, No. 2, pp. 299-314.

[57] Drucker, H., Cortes, C., Jackel, L.D., LeCun, Y., Vapnik, V. (1994). Boosting and other ensemble methods. *Neural Computation*, Vol. 6, No. 6, pp. 1289-1301.

[58] Jacobs, R.A., Jordan, M.I., Nowlan, S.J., Hinton, G.E. (1991). Adaptive mixtures of local experts. *Neural Computation*, Vol. 3, No. 1, pp. 79-87.

[59] Jordan, M.J., Jacobs, R.A. (1994). Hierarchical mixtures of experts and the EM algorithm. *Neural Computation*, Vol. 6, No. 2, pp. 181-214

[60] Schapire, R.E. (1990). The strength of weak learnability. *Machine Learning*, Vol. 5, No. 2, pp. 197-227.

[61] Drucker, H., Schapire, R., Simard, P. (1993). Boosting performance in neural networks. *Int. J. Pattern Recognition Artif. Intelligence*, Vol. 7, No. 4, pp. 704-709.

[62] Dam, H.H., Abbass, H.A., Lokan, C., Yao, X. (2008). Neural-Based Learning Classifier Systems. *IEEE Transactions on Knowledge and Data Engineering*, Vol. 20, No. 1, pp. 26-39.

[63] Suárez Araujo, C.P., García Báez, P., Sánchez Rodríguez , A., Santana Rodríguez, J.J. (2009). HUMANN-based system to determine pesticides using multifluorescence spectra: An ensemble approach. *Analytical and Bioanalytical Chemistry*, Vol. 394, No. 4, pp. 1059-1072.

[64] García Báez, P., Suárez Araujo, C.P., Sánchez Rodríguez, Á., Santana Rodríguez, J.J. (2010). Towards an efficient computational method for fluorescence identification of fungicides using data fusion and neural ensemble techniques. *Luminescence*, in press.

[65] Roli, F., Giadnto, G. (2002). Design of multiple classifier systems, In: *Hybrid Methods in Pattern Recognition*, Bunke, H., Kandel, A. (Ed.), pp. 199-226, World Scientific Publishing, Singapore.

[66] Ruta, D., Gabrys, D. (2005). Classifier selection for majority voting. *Information Fusion*, Vol. 6, No. 1, pp. 63-81.

[67] Folstein, M.F., Folstein, S.E., McHugh, P.R. (1975). Mini-mental state". A practical method for grading the cognitive state of patients for the clinician. *Journal of psychiatric research*, Vol. 12, No. 3, pp. 189-198.

[68] Reisberg, B. (1988). Functional Assessment Staging (FAST). *Psychopharmacology Bulletin*, Vol. 24, pp. 653-659.

[69] Katz, S.C., Ford, A.B., Moskowitz, R.W. (1963). Studies of illness in the aged. The index of ADL: a standardized measure of biological and psychosocial function. *JAMA*, Vol. 185, pp. 914-919.

[70] Mahoney, F.I., Barthel, D. (1965). Functional evaluation: The Barthel Index. *Maryland State Medical Journal*, Vol. 14, pp. 61-65.

[71] Lawton, M.P., Brody, E.M. (1969). Assessment of older people: self-mantaining and instrumental activities of daily living. *Gerontologist*, Vol. 9, pp. 179-186.

[72] Yamaguchi, S., Tsuchiya, H., Yamagata, S., Toyoda, G., Kobayashi, S. (2000). Event-related brain potentials in response to novel sounds in dementia. *Clinical Neurophysiology*, Vol. 111, pp. 195-203.

[73] Jansen, B.H., Allam, A., Kota, P., Lachance, K., Osho, A., Sundaresan, K. (2004). An exploratory study of factors affecting single trial P300 detection. *IEEE Transactions on Biomedical Engineering*, Vol. 51, pp. 975-978.

[74] Polikar, R., Udpa, L., Udpa, S.S., Honavar, V. (2001). Learn++: an incremental learning algorithm for supervised neural networks. *IEEE Transactions on Systems, Man and Cybernetics*, Vol. 31, pp. 497-508.

[75] Horn, J.F., Habert, M.O., Kas, A., Malek, Z., Maksud, P., Lacomblez, L., Giron, A., Fertil, B. (2009). Differential automatic diagnosis between Alzheimer's disease and frontotemporal dementia based on perfusion SPECT images. *Artificial Intelligence in Medicine*, Vol. 47, No. 2, pp. 147-158.

[76] Tzourio-Mazoyer, N., Landeau, B., Papathanassiou, D., Crivello, F., Etard, O., Delcroix, N. et al. (2002). Automated anatomical labeling of activations in SPM using a macroscopic anatomical parcellation of the MNI MRI single-subject brain. *Neuroimage*, Vol. 15, No. 1, pp. 273-289.

[77] McCullagh, P., Nelder, J.A. (1994). An interpretation of partial least squares. *Journal of American Statistical Association*, Vol. 89, No. 425, pp. 122-127.

[78] Cortes, C., Vapnik, V. (1995). Support-vector networks. *Machine Learning*, Vol. 20, No. 3, pp. 273-297.

In: Alzheimer's Diagnosis   ISBN: 978-1-61209-846-3
Editor: Charles E. Ronson, pp. 137-174   ©2011 Nova Science Publishers, Inc.

Chapter VII

Milestones and Difficulties in Alzheimer's Disease Diagnosis

Lucia Picchi, Marco Vista and Monica Mazzoni
Alzheimer Diagnostic Unit, Section of Neurology, Campo
di Marte Hospital, Lucca, Italy

Progressive aging of population will make Alzheimer's Disease (AD) one of the most important health problems of the next years, challenging social security and health systems of industrialized countries. The present work analyzes the resources and the difficulties of the diagnostic flow charts in territorial reality where more important space is given to the clinical activity rather than to research. When first symptoms of a possible dementia appear, people contact general practioner, directly or pushed by their relatives. The general practioner is very important for the screening in case of a possible dementia because his/her attention and sensibility make early diagnosis possible. General practioner, in fact, usually requires a consult to the specialist (neurologist, psychiatric, geriatrician), which, working in équipe with the psychologist, can begin a multi-dimentional evaluation of first level that includes: 1) medical history; 2) general and neurological examination; 3) neuropsychological screening; 4) evaluation of functional abilities; 5) assessment of patient's relationship and family context; 6) routine and specific blood tests; 7) at least one neuroimaging exam (e.g. CT scan). Undoubtedly, the results of the clinical and instrumental investigations may provide useful elements for the differential diagnosis of dementia and, therefore, for adequate medical, psychological and socio-relational caring. However, the diagnostic process remains, to date, a puzzle that clinicians build progressively due to the lack of specific biomarkers.

1. Background

Dementia is an umbrella term that describes a chronic or progressive impairment of cognitive functions of the brain such as memory, language, gnosis, praxis, and executive functions. It may also be accompanied by disturbances of mood, behavior and personality (the so called Behavioral and Psychological Symptoms of Dementia, BPSD). All these symptoms are supposed to interfere with normal activities of daily life [1]. This condition is not a natural consequence of aging, but is due to pathologic processes affecting the brain, which are caused by a number of diseases such as Alzheimer's Disease (AD), Dementia with Lewy bodies (DLB), Fronto-Temporal Dementia (FTD) and so on [2]. AD is responsible for the majority of cases [2]. However, aging is considered the major risk factor: although there are cases of dementia described in people before the age of 65, data from epidemiologic studies suggest that the chance of developing dementia after the age of 65 doubles every five years [3]. With the increase in longevity, dementia will be a huge global problem, which every department of health and human services in the world will have to cope with.

The enormous significance of this problem is coming from epidemiologic data: it has been assessed that there are 35.6 million people living with dementia worldwide in 2010, increasing to 65.7 million by 2030 and 115.4 million by 2050 [4]. The cost of dementia represents a heavy burden to society, estimated at 604 billion dollars in 2010, which accounts for around 1% of the world's gross domestic product (considering *dementia care* as a country, it would be the world's 18th largest economy, ranking between Turkey and Indonesia) [4]. This amount should be equally divided between informal care and direct costs of social care in the proportion of 42%, while direct medical care costs are at 16% [4]. 70% of global costs occurred in Western Europe and North America, while the prevalence of dementia in these two areas is around 45% [4]. In Europe, the annual cost is estimated at 141 billion euros [5]. Costs per person are about 32,865 dollars in high income countries [4], which is about 21,000 euros in Europe [5]: all these costs are expected to increase in the next future.

On these assumptions, the diagnosis of dementia is greatly significant as for the handling of such a multifaceted disease, not only affecting the ill person, but also the whole of his/her family, with a striking impact on the their life from the disclosure of the diagnosis to the patient's death.

From the start, it is usually a relative who recognizes a change in the behavior of the patient, and it is only rarely that a patient complains of a memory decline. Afterwards, the more frequent conduct is to ask to a general practitioner for medical advice. Since then, the diagnostic work-up starts: general health care providers should be able to meet the needs of people fearing dementia and ensure a professional approach to this particular demand.

The aim of this paper is to define simple but specific proceedings enabling clinicians to diagnose dementia, to be used in local settings with limited resources, such as general practitioners or specialized physicians in peripheral hospitals. Among the different forms of dementia, AD is the most frequent [4, 6] and, on this account, the clinical pattern of this disease will be examined more exhaustively. With today's techniques and practices, these aims seem to be enough for practical purpose, since therapies are only symptomatic (even if some pharmacological studies suggest that the current available treatments are not as effective in stemming cognitive decline if the starting is delayed [7]), and early diagnosis is most needed for decision making and advanced planning.

The main target is to help patients' families in managing the disease from all perspectives, such as improving individual autonomy in daily living activities, reducing the need for informal care, coping with BPSD - which are the most important causes of the caregivers' burdens and the patients' institutionalizations - and also beginning to endure power of attorney and guardianship, addressing safety concerns about living alone and driving ability, providing caregivers with detailed information about the disease, and then, ultimately, improving the quality of life of the patient as well as of his/her family [1].

Unfortunately, owing to the current worldwide financial crisis, health and human services have to account for every asset or resource they use in order to optimize medical activities: keeping this in mind, it is our primary interest to identify all the single, specific steps allowing us to reach a diagnosis avoiding economic waste.

2. The Diagnosis of Dementia

The diagnosis of dementia is a clinical process taking into account several symptoms and signs, and excluding other causes. The diagnostic work-up is based upon criteria sets to increase the accuracy and reliability of the diagnosis. In recent years, groups of experts convened to establish criteria based on personal experience and scientific data: at the beginning, they established dementia criteria (see Tab.1), then, they outlined specific criteria for each of the different disorders, as distinguishing features of various forms of dementia have been fully recognized thanks to the progresses of scientific knowledge about clinic, histopathology, molecular biology and genetics (see Tab.2). For their significance, due to epidemiology and to the interest raised within the scientific community and in public opinion, AD criteria are numerous (see Tab.3 and Tab.4), highly detailed, and eventually revised with years (see Tab.5 and Tab.6). Moreover, Neurological Scientific Societies in many countries set up task forces to develop Guidelines for the diagnosis and the management of dementia, in particular for AD [8-10]. The diagnostic work-up has been well defined, obtained the consensus of all the attending experts, and the scientific evidence of every step was, as usually, assessed according to levels of certainty (classes of evidence) and recommendations are graded based on the strength of the evidence.

Table 1. ICD-10 Criteria for Dementia [82]

1.	Evidence of each of the following:
a.	A decline in memory, which is most evident in the learning of new information, although in more severe cases, the recall of previously learned information may be also affected. The impairment applies to both verbal and non-verbal material. The decline should be objectively verified by obtaining a reliable history from an informant, supplemented, if possible, by neuropsychological tests or quantified cognitive assessments.
b.	A decline in other cognitive abilities characterized by deterioration in judgment and thinking, such as planning and organizing, and in the general processing of information. Evidence for this should be obtained when possible from interviewing an informant, supplemented, if possible, by neuropsychological tests or quantified objective assessments. Deterioration from a previously higher level of performance should be established.
2.	Preserved awareness of the environment (i.e. absence of clouding of consciousness) during a period of time long enough to enable the unequivocal demonstration of symptoms in 1. When there are superimposed episodes of delirium the diagnosis of dementia should be deferred.
3.	A decline in emotional control or motivation, or a change in social behavior, manifest as at least one of the following: • emotional lability; • irritability; • apathy; • coarsening of social behavior.
4.	For a confident clinical diagnosis, the symptoms in 1 should have been present for at least six months; if the period since the manifest onset is shorter, the diagnosis can only be tentative.

Table 2. Diagnostic criteria of major neurodegenerative dementias

Disease	Criteria	Bibliography
AD	National Institute for Neurologic Disorders and Stroke- Alzheimer's Disease related Associations (NINCDS-ADRDA)	McKhann et al., 1984 [11]
		Dubois et al., 2007 [35]
	Research criteria for the diagnosis of AD	McKhann et al., 2010 [83]
	Criteria for AD dementia	Alafuzoff et al., 2006 [84]
	BrainNet Europe Consortium	Braak & Braak, 1991 [85]
	Braak & Braak	1997 [86]
	Regan Institute CERAD	Mirra et al., 1991 [87]
DLB	Consortium on DLB International Workshop	McKeith et al., 1996 [88]
	Second DLB International Workshop	McKeith et al., 1999 [89]
	Third DLB International Workshop	McKeith et al., 2005 [90]
FTD	Lund-Manchester criteria	Brun et al., 1994 [91]
	Consensus criteria	Neary at al., 1998 [92]
	Consortium for FTLD	McKhann et al., 2001 [93]
		Cairns et al., 2007 [94]
PD-D		Braak et al., 2004 [95]
	Movement Disorders task force	Emre et al., 2007 [96]
PSP	NINDS-SPSP	Hauw et al., 1994 [97]
		Litvan et al., 1996 [98]
CBD		Boeve et al., 1999 [99]
		Riley et al., 2000 [100]
	Office of Rare Diseases	Dickson at al., 2002 [101]

AD= Alzheimer's disease; DLB= Dementia with Lewy bodies; FTD= Fronto-Temporal Dementia; PD-D= Parkinson's Disease Dementia; PSP= Progressive Supranuclear Plasy; CBD= Corticobasal Degeneration

Table 3. DSM-IV criteria for Alzheimer's Disease [102]

A.	Alzheimer's disease is characterized by progressive decline and ultimately loss of multiple cognitive functions, including both:
a.	Memory impairment: impaired ability to learn new information or to recall previously learned information.
b.	And at least one of the following:
i.	Loss of word comprehension ability, for example, inability to respond to "Your daughter is on the phone." (aphasia)
ii.	Loss of ability to perform complex tasks involving muscle coordination, for example, bathing or dressing (apraxia)
iii.	Loss of ability to recognize and use familiar objects, for example, clothing (agnosia);
iv.	Loss of ability to plan, organize, and execute normal activities, for example, going shopping.
B.	The problems in "A" represent a substantial decline from previous abilities and cause significant problems in everyday functioning.
C.	The problems in "A" begin slowly and gradually become more severe.
D.	The problems in "A" are not due to:
a.	Other conditions that cause progressive cognitive decline, among them: stroke, Parkinson's disease, Huntington's chorea, brain tumor, etc.
b.	Other conditions that cause dementia, among them: hypothyroidism, HIV infection, syphilis, and deficiencies in niacin, vitamin B12, and folic acid.
E.	The problems in "A" are not caused by episodes of delirium.
F.	The problems in "A" are not caused by another mental illness: depression, schizophrenia, etc.

Table 4. NINCDS-ADRDA Criteria for clinical diagnosis of Alzheimer's Disease [11]

Criteria for diagnosis of **Probable** Alzheimer's Disease: • Dementia established by clinical examination, and documented by a standard test of cognitive function (e.g. Mini-Mental State Examination, Blessed Dementia Scale, etc.), and confirmed by neuropsychological tests. • Significant deficiencies in two or more areas of cognition, for example, word comprehension and task-completion ability. • Progressive deterioration of memory and other cognitive functions. • No loss of consciousness. • Onset from age 40 to 90, typically after 65. • No other diseases or disorders that could account for the loss of memory and cognition.

A diagnosis of Probable Alzheimer's Disease is supported by:
• Progressive deterioration of specific cognitive functions: language (aphasia), motor skills (apraxia), and perception (agnosia).
• Impaired activities of daily living and altered patterns of behavior.
• A family history of similar problems, particularly if confirmed by neurological testing.
• The following laboratory results:
  o Normal cerebrospinal fluid (lumbar puncture test).
  o Normal electroencephalogram (EEG) test of brain activity.
  o Evidence of cerebral atrophy in a series of CT scans.

Other features consistent with Alzheimer's Disease • Plateaus in the course of illness progression. • CT findings normal for the person's age. • Associated symptoms, including: depression, insomnia, incontinence, delusions, hallucinations, weight loss, sex problems, and significant verbal, emotional, and physical outbursts. • Other neurological abnormalities, especially in advanced disease: including: increased muscle tone and a shuffling gait.
Features that decrease the likelihood of Alzheimer's Disease: • Sudden onset. • Such early symptoms as: seizures, gait problems, and loss of vision and coordination.
Clinical diagnosis of **Possible** Alzheimer's Disease: • May be made on the basis of the dementia syndrome, in the absence of other neurologic, psychiatric, or systemic disorders sufficient to cause dementia, and in the presence of variations in the onset, in the presentation, or in the clinical course. • May be made in the presence of a second systemic or brain disorder sufficient to produce dementia, which is not considered to be the cause of the dementia; and • Should be used in research studies when a single, gradually progressive severe cognitive deficit is identified in the absence of other identifiable cause.

In recent years, the process of the diagnosis of dementia evolved based on new scientific knowledge and a lot of diagnostic tools are now available. However, no specific biomarker has yet been recognized as absolute, but a puzzle of more markers is needed in order to reach a probabilistic certainty of diagnosis. On the basis of these clinical criteria, it is possible to make an *in vivo* diagnosis: as a matter of fact, a definite diagnosis of dementia needs both clinical criteria and histopathologic evidence obtained through biopsy or autopsy [11].

Table 5. Proposed research diagnostic criteria for Alzheimer's Disease [35]

Probable AD: A plus one or more supportive features B, C, D or E: A. Presence of an early and significant episodic memory impairment that is gradual and progressive , reported by patients or informants over more than 6 months, isolated or associated with other cognitive changes at the onset of AD or as AD advances: objective evidence of significantly impaired episodic memory on testing, that generally consists of recall deficit that does not improve significantly or does not normalize with cueing or recognition testing and after effective encoding of information has been previously controlled
Supportive features: B. Structural neuroimaging (proven medial temporal lobe atrophy with specific neuroradiological methods such as voxel based morphometry) C. Lumbar puncture (low amyloid β1-42, increased total tau or phosphor-tau concentration) D. Functional neuroimaging with PET (reduced regional glucose metabolism or positivity with amyloid ligands) E. Genetic
Exclusion criteria from medical history and clinical features

Clinicians should apply these flow charts to merely reach a well supported diagnosis: firstly, the aim is to diagnose the presence of dementia, secondly, we need to find its cause, by distinguishing between primary degenerative disorders and forms of dementias which are secondary to other diseases, and which sometimes could be reversible. But this two-step procedure is not easily applicable, because it is not always possible to use all the suggestions from the guidelines, since clinical settings greatly vary depending on the accessibility to specific diagnostic tools, which in some cases are very expensive or invasive. On this assumption, the following paragraphs include a review of recent clinical guidelines for the diagnosis of dementia, and the minimum diagnostic work-up is outlined in the simplest way, so that each physician would be able to perform it in any kind of clinical settings by means of easily accessible resources.

Table 6. Operational Research Criteria for Alzheimer's Disease [83]

Clinical criteria for the diagnosis of AD dementia
•   Insidious onset (over months to years)
•   Clear-cut history of worsening of cognition by report or observation
•   Cognitive deficits in one of the two categories:
1. Amnestic presentation
2. Non-amnestic presentation:
i. Language (word finding)
ii. Visual ability (object agnosia, prosopoagnosia, simultanagnosia or alexia)
iii. Executive function (impaired reasoning, judgment, problem solving)
iv. [deficits in other cognitive domains should be present]
Clinical characterization for AD dementia
1. *Probable* AD dementia
Meets clinical criteria for AD and without evidence of any alternative diagnoses (in particular, no significant cerebrovascular disease); this could be enhanced by one of the following features:
a. Documented decline (based on interview of informants or cognitive testing)
b. Biomarker positive
i. Low CSF $A\beta_{1-42}$, incremented total or phospho-tau
ii. Positive amyloid PET imaging
iii. Decreased FDG uptake on PET in temporoparietal cortex
c. Proven atrophy on structural MR in specific regions
d. Mutation carrier (PSEN1, PSEN2, APP)
2. *Possible* AD dementia
a. Atypical course
b. Biomarkers obtained and negative
c. Mixed presentation (cerebrovascular disease)

2.1. Clinical History

When assessing a demented person, a focused clinical history is fundamental and, as many experts stated [12-13], the diagnosis could already be suspected on the mere reporting of the patient's daily living. A well performed interview would give the chance to achieve precious information about everyday life carried out with the interference of cognitive impairment and its consequences on personal and social activities. Since dementia is characterized by a cognitive deficit and lack of awareness of their own difficulties, the interview should be conducted both with the patient and an informant, usually a relative, who plays the role of the *primary caregiver*, that is the figure more involved in the process of informal caregiving, usually the patient's spouse or son/daughter; more rarely other relatives or formal caregivers, the latter could be both working at the patients' home or in a nursing home. This relationship is so deep that this disease affects the patient as well as the caregiver, so that it is usually referred to as a "*dyad*".

The interview is split into two parts: during the first, the examiner speaks both with the patient and the caregiver, but during the second, the two interviews are conducted separately. Also, from the very beginning of the first part of the interview, the physician shall identifies a typical behavior: the patients are usually unable to remember even their own birthday or the job of their whole life, while place of birth and schooling are less frequently lost. When patients are in difficulties, they often turn to their caregiver. Sometimes patients themselves complain of subjective loss of memory but, more often, they deny every such complaint reported by their caregivers, and this sometimes unleashes agitation and irritability, and even violent reactions. The course of dementia involves the patients' progressive loss of ability to identify deficits resulting from their disease; anosognosia shows with the following symptoms: inadequate awareness of behavioral alterations, changes of personality, dishinibition, and affective deficit; wrong causal attribution of memory and cognitive deficits; underestimation of the limitations in daily living activities due to the illness, and proneness to maintain habits and behaviors without adopting compensatory strategies, with consequent adoption of risky behaviors; explicit and verbal non-acknowledgement of being affected with a pathological process, and descriptions of an unchanged self compared with that previous to the illness. These are common characteristics of anosognosia which, however, manifests itself with distinctive and peculiar features based on the different forms of dementia. In AD, the loss of awareness usually appears later, and more gradually, as the frontal lobes are damaged after the parietal lobes [14]. By asking patients about their past and current health problems, the examiner may get the idea of the level of cognitive impairment and the insight of disease. As far as the unawareness of the illness is concerned, it is difficult to succeed in identifying the right tools to be used to objectively assess it and give it a measure. In time, with the increasing interest about anosognosia, several questionnaires to assess awareness have been formulated, including a cross-comparison between the subjects' description of their own cognitive abilities and the objective performance in neuropsychological tests; or between the subjects' description of themselves in multiple areas of their daily life (cognitive, functional, behavioral), and the caregivers' description of the patients [15]. In the first case, the comparison is between "subjective" – the patient's self-ratings – and "objective" – the neuropsychological tests scores – data, while in the second case, we have a comparison between two absolutely "subjective" data, affected by the personal characteristics both of the patients and the caregivers [16-18]; the Deficits Identification Questionnaire (DIQ) is one of the scales that applies to this last approach [19, 20].

The examiner must pay attention to the patient's language, which can be characterized by anomias, that is the use of "passé-partout" words ("thing", "that", and so on), paraphasias and circumlocutions, and by auditory verbal comprehension impairment. The memory of old facts, mostly autobiographical, is well preserved, while recent events are forgotten. Sometimes motor behavior is impaired with praxis deficits, such as difficulties in using a pen or taking off one's coat; more rarely, the patients show an impairment in reaching an object handed them by the examiner (a sign included in Balint's syndrome).

The mood is to be addressed too, carefully evaluating all the aspects of depression and anxiety. There is often an overlapping between dementia and depression, the last could mimic dementia at the onset showing impaired memory and concentration. Awareness is still preserved in depression, and patients with depression probably complain about memory disturbances more than demented persons. The differential diagnosis is still difficult, but a deep neuropsychological evaluation can be considerably helpful. Behavior is one of the most sensible keys to address a suspect of diagnosis: inhibited or apathetic behavior is more typical of AD, while uninhibited or talkative behavior is typical of FTD.

Recording the patient's history from the caregiver is as much important: an independent informant may provide a fundamental supplement of information about the patient's current condition and symptoms, about cognitive functions and their influence on activities in everyday life and behavioral and psychological symptoms. The caregivers, knowing the patient long before the disease, have the sensibility to notice even the subtlest changes from earlier life. Living with the patient, they are also able to describe the symptoms in detail, having witnessed for a long time. However, there are some traps in giving great importance to the caregivers' report in our clinical history: the results may depend on the extent and quality of the dyad-relationship, on the emotional state and the personality traits of the caregivers [21]. Personality stands for the whole set of faculties, attitudes, and qualities that allows us to tell individuals apart [22]. Personality traits assume an important role as far as the subjective perception of the stress is concerned. The definition of stress in itself implies all that, as it is meant to be the mechanism connecting subjective-internal elaboration and objective-external event. As personality traits are implicated in the process of elaboration of the stressors, and therefore in the level of stress, they also necessarily affect the state of health. Within the family context in which it manifests itself, dementia undoubtedly represents an important factor of stress, which affects primary caregivers. On this account, it seems worthwhile to assess the role of personality in caregivers, emerging during the process of caregiving. Particularly, there have to be some personality traits which are to some extent defensive against stress or, otherwise, caregivers will be more vulnerable to it. Furthermore, a psychologist assessing patient's relationships and family contexts would be of great value in order to set a behavioral rehabilitation enabling the patients to improve their functional capabilities and avoid pharmacological intervention to treat BPSD. Unfortunately, a multi-disciplinary team including neurologist/geriatrician/psychiatrist, and a psychologist, that should be considered a gold standard, is also very expensive and it is a scarcely available resource. Moreover, a significant number of demented people do not have a reliable caregiver.

2.2. Physical and Neurological Examination

The general physical examination is intended to ascertain whether there are significant co-morbidities, which may be the cause of, or contribute to, cognitive symptoms: reversible dementia could be a condition in all the most important organ failures, like chronic heart failure, chronic obstructive pulmonary disease, hepatic encephalopathy, renal failure with chronic anemia, electrolytes disorders. Hypothyroidism and, rarely, other endocrinal diseases are characterized by mental deterioration. Deficiency of vitamin B_{12} is the most frequent hypovitaminosis associated to impairment of cognitive performance and low blood level of folic acid is often present in demented people, but that is not the cause of dementia; not rarely, alcoholism is the cause of bad nutrition, with a scarce intake of vitamin B_1, that may be the cause of an acute Wernicke syndrome or a chronic Korsakoff's syndrome. In all cancer patients with cognitive impairment, a paraneoplastic encephalopathy must be addressed. An infectious disease should be suspected when there is fever; however, every time the anamnesis and the course of mental deterioration arise specific hypothesis, selected tests should be carried out (HIV, TB, syphilis, B. burgdorferi, etc.). Finally, a detailed anamnesis of all the drugs taken by the patient should be carried out in order to ascertain if an iatrogenic cause could reduce the patient's mental efficiency.

It is important to focus on neurosensorial impairment, especially visual and acoustic, which can oversize possible cognitive disturbances due to sensory deprivation. Visual deficit and/or hearing loss could interfere with neuropsychological assessment, making our results doubtful with the risk of overrating them.

An abrupt onset of the symptoms must arouse the suspicion of a delirium, that is, by definition, acute, occurring from several hours to several days, but that is distinguished from dementia by the impairment of sensorium. Patients with delirium show fluctuations of consciousness with impaired attention and concentration. However, demented people are at high risk of delirium and these two disorders overlap, particularly during hospitalization. Delirium very often constitutes a step-wise deterioration, probably unmasking incipient or pre-existing dementia.

An exhaustive neurological examination in early dementia is significant in order to identify the typical signs of the different forms of degenerative diseases and differentiate them from other pathologies which affect the central nervous system. To this end, examiners should evaluate the presence of extrapyramidal signs: in this case, the Parkinson's Disease Dementia (PD-D) or one of the parkinsonisms with dementia, such as DLB, could be evoked; in order to distinguish between PD-D and DLB, the *1-year rule* has been established: if motor signs anticipate mental deterioration for 12 months, then PD-D diagnosis is more reliable; otherwise, in case of concurrent extrapyramidal signs and dementia onsets, DLB must be suspected. Parkinsonisms with dementia are well described and their clinical criteria are widely detailed (see Tab. 2). Some signs and symptoms are peculiar of different diseases: visual hallucinations and fluctuating cognition are core symptoms of DLB, while REM sleep behavior disorder and severe neuroleptic sensitivity constitute suggestive features; if vertical or horizontal gaze is impaired and in presence of postural instability with unexpected falls and dysarthria, a Progressive Supranuclear Palsy (PSP) must be suspected; where extrapyramidal signs are clearly lateralized, a Corticobasal Degeneration

(CBD) should be diagnosed, particularly in presence of ideomotor apraxia or alien hand syndrome; at last, normal pressure hydrocephalus (NPH) must be kept in mind, as it is one of the few causes of reversible dementia, which is characterized by the triad 'mental deterioration, gait impairment and urinary incontinence'.

When lateralizing signs are detected, a vascular damage should be addressed, and space-occupying intracranial lesions (i.e., tumors, subdural hematoma), inflammatory or toxic-metabolic diseases must be taken in account. An abrupt onset is more likely present in cerebrovascular disease.

Primitive reflexes such as palmar grasp or palmomental reflexes could be the signs of a frontal lobes dysfunction (frontal release signs), often found in AD, as well as in FTD. Decreased olfactory sense is another frequent feature in demented people, as well as parietal sensory signs and gait disorders, but they are less specific to a particular form of dementia.

2.3. Lab Tests

Routine blood tests are necessary as a base for differential diagnosis (to rule out reversible dementias) and in order to indentify co-morbidities. No specific tests are necessary, but usually a basic screening includes a complete blood cell count, glucose, renal and liver function, electrolytes, calcium, thyroid hormones, Vitamin B_{12} and folic acid. Tests for syphilis and HIV must be considered in selected cases with high risk factors or suggestive clinical features. Omocysteine is described as an important risk factor in ischemic vascular brain damage, but also in AD [23]. Other lab tests must be taken into account based on particular diagnostic hypotheses.

2.4. Neuropsychological Testing

The assessment of cognitive impairment is an essential part for the clinical evaluation of dementia, even if it is time consuming. Screening tests (see Tab.7) to detect and grossly quantify mental deterioration have been developed [24]: they can be useful to objectify, although roughly, an impaired performance, obtaining a score in order to compare it to standardized data of a '*normal*' population. Although it may give the false impression to have the absolute data, a screening neuropsychological test is however useful, because it provides an index for evaluating the actual mental status of the patient, giving the idea of the severity of the impairment and allowing a follow up in time. In these last years, many relatively brief screening tests have been proposed, but only the Mini-mental State Examination (MMSE) [25] is the most commonly used world-wide. Lots of studies reported its shortcomings [26-28], suggesting variations or alternatives (see Tab. 7), but it is clear that MMSE is still the best available, even with its many limitations, and every clinician, with a good know-how, is able to use this tool at best, not only for a quantitative, but also for a qualitative judgment. The cut-off below 24/30, after the age and education corrections, which is considered as pathological, is only a starting point: it is clear that with a score below 18, the likelihood of dementia presence is high, while with a score over 26, the absence of dementia is very likely. Middle scores are inconclusive. The annual rate of decrease is stated on the average of 3.4 points, but it largely varies [29]. MMSE was developed for AD, and it is not the best tool for assessing other forms of dementia, because it lacks in testing language, visual-spatial skills and executive function. However, it is also recommended in the guidelines for the diagnosis of Parkinson's Disease Dementia [30], using some sub-items (repeatedly subtract 7 starting at 100 for attention, copy two overlapping pentagons for visual-constructive ability and free recall of three words for memory).

A lot of other screening tests have been developed (see Tab. 7) with the aim to achieve both high sensitivity and specificity, for the early diagnosis of cognitive impairment too, which in recent literature has been one of the most controversial matter of discussion [31]: the symptomatic pre-dementia, defined as Mild Cognitive Impairment (MCI) is a syndrome that cannot be diagnosed through a lab test, as it needs a clinical judgment based on clinical cognitive and functional criteria as well as dementia. MCI has been recently re-defined as a change in cognition with impairment in one or more cognitive domains and preservation of independence in functional abilities [32]. Lower performance in one or more cognitive domains should be demonstrated by means of some neuropsychological assessments (better when repeated examinations are available, showing a decline in performance over time). These cognitive changes must be mild, that is they should not interfere with social and occupational functioning, as the judgment is to be tailored on the individuals themselves: obviously, a 60-years old manager should be assessed in a different way compared to a 80-years old housekeeper. MCI, like dementia, can be due to different etiologies, and we need biomarkers to distinguish MCI associated to AD from other forms (new Criteria for MCI due to AD have been recently proposed) [33].

Table 7. Some of the screening tests available in the literature

Test <10 minutes	Bibliography	Sensitivity	Specificity
Six Item Screener	Callahan et al., 2002[103]	88.7%	88%
Clock Drawing	Lee et al., 1996 [104]	67%	97%
3-Word Recall	Cullum CM et al., 1993 [105]	65%	85%
Mini-Cog	Borson S, 2000 [106]	76%	89%
Memory Impairment Screen	Bushke H et al., 1999 [107]	80%	96%
Brief Alzheimer Screen	Mendiondo MS et al., 2003 [108]	99%	87%
AD8	Galvin EJ et al, 2005 [109]	74-85%	86%
General Practioner Assessment of Cognition	Brodaty H et al, 2002 [110]	85%	86%
Blessed Orientation Memory Concentration Test	Katzman R et al., 1993 [111]	88%	94%
Hopkins Verbal Learning Test-Revised	Brandt & Benedict, 2001 [112]	87%	98%
Abbreviated Mental Test	Hodkinson HM, 1972 [113]	96%	80%
Informant Questionnaire for Cognitive Decline in the Elderly	Jorm AF, 2004 [114]	79-100%	68-86%
7-min	Solomon et al., 1998 [115]	93%	93%
Short Test of Mental Status	Kokemen et al., 1987 [116]	86-92%	91-93%
Time and Change Test	Inouye et al., 1998 [117]	63%	96%
Mental Alternation Test	Jones et al., 1993 [118]	95%	81%
Telephone Interview for Cognitive Status	Brandt et al., 1988 [119]	82,4-100%	83-87%
Test >10 minutes	**Bibliography**	**Sensitivity**	**Specificity**
Mini Mental State Examination	Folstein et al., 1975 [25]	80-85%	76-80%
Addenbrooke's Cognitive Examination	Mioshi et al., 2006 [120]	94%	89%
Montreal Cognitive Assessment	Nasreddine et al., 2005 [121]	90%	90%
Mattis Dementia Rating Scale	Rascovsky et al., 2008 [122]	85%	85%
CERAD Battery	Chandler et al., 2005 [123]	80%	81%
Neurobehavioral Cognitive Status Examination	Kiernan et al., 1987 [124]	100%	83%
Short Cognitive Evaluation Battery	Robert PH et al., 2003 [125]	93.8%	85%
Rowland Universal Dementia Assessment Scale	Storey et al., 2004 [126]	89%	98%
Short and Sweet Interview for Dementia	Belle et al., 2000 [127]	94%	91%
Functional Activities Questionnaire	Pfeffer et al., 1982 [128]	80%	87%
Modified Mini Mental State Examination	Bland & Newman, 2001 [129]	88%	90%
Cognitive Assessment Screening test	Drachman et al., 1996 [130]	95%	88%
Cambridge Cognitive Examination	Roth et al., 1988 [131]	88%	75%
Community Screening Interview for Dementia	Hall et al., 2000 [132]	87%	83.1%
Dementia Questionnaire	Silverman et al., 1986 [133]	89%	72%

Although the screening tests are useful as they indicate when a person is no longer normal, a detailed assessment is needed in any case. A second level neuropsychological assessment with batteries composed of several tests specifically designed to outline the deficits in different cognitive domains is required not only to satisfy the clinical criteria for dementia, but also because, in their early stages, all the main forms of dementia have a selective anatomical localization, reflecting some typical patterns of neuropsychological impairment. This allows clinicians to speculate the nature of the pathogenesis of the clinical syndrome. Unfortunately, no specific neuropsychological patterns were found yet within the available post-mortem proven studies [34].

A battery of neuropsychological tests should be able to evaluate the language, memory, attention and executive functions, praxis and visual-spatial abilities. Memory impairment is considered the core trait of dementia and should be systematically assessed. Several neuropsychological studies tried to highlight peculiar aspects of memory impairment in different forms and stages of dementia. The testing of episodic memory allows to identify an early deficit, discriminating between healthy controls and demented persons, particularly with a delayed recall testing [35]. Moreover, to identify AD, a specificity has been found through the use of paradigms of cued recall, which allows to assess the effective encoding after the semantic cueing which usually maximize the retrieval: healthy controls, as well as non-AD patients (PD-D, and so on), are discriminated from AD patients with a sensitivity and specificity of 93% to 99% [36]. Healthy controls and non-AD patients, whose deficits in delayed recall could be attributed to attentional deficits or inefficient strategies, are helped by semantic cueing, that is inefficient for AD patients, because of their raw impairment of encoding and storage processes. This typical trait of memory impairment has been recently included among the core diagnostic criteria for AD proposed for the relevant scientific research (see Tab.5 and 6). A semantic memory testing, a cognitive dominion overlapping memory and language, is essential to distinguish AD from Semantic Dementia, a phenotypic syndrome which belongs to FTD. Executive dysfunction is typical of frontal or subcortical lesions, while language, praxis and visual-spatial functions are more involved when the damage affects particular areas of the brain cortex.

Several complete neuropsychological batteries have been proposed world-wide, such as the Geriatric Mental State Examination [37], the Cambridge Examination for Mental Disorder of the Elderly (CAMDEX), including the CAMCOG [38], the Alzheimer's Disease Assessment Scale (ADAS), including the ADAS-Cog [39] and so on. Only in Italy, there are many batteries based on neuropsychological grounds and formalized with an advanced statistical analyses: the Milano Overall Dementia Assessment

(MODA) [40], the Italian study on dementia battery (SMID) [41], and the Mental Deterioration Battery (MDB) [42-44]. Furthermore, each neuropsychological lab usually creates its own battery using the more sensitive tests available in literature, in order to have flexible tools covering most of the domains and customizable for all types of dementia. The second level neuropsychological testing should ideally be performed by trained psychologists in adequate settings; this condition is not always easily accessible by all the clinicians and expensive; it adds no fundamental information to the change management of dementia, but it offers an incomparable help to differential diagnosis and increases sensitivity in early diagnosis.

2.5. Assessing ADLs (Activities of Daily Living)

The cognitive impairment is supposed to interfere with the patient's activities of daily living (ADLs) so that we can consider the condition of the patient as a dementia: of course, assessing ADLs becomes a necessary step in the diagnostic work-up. Semi-structured interviews are usually used to evaluate ADLs, and different areas could be investigated. Eating, dressing, washing, etc. are basic activities of daily living (BADLs), usually impaired in more advanced phases of dementia. Instrumental activities of daily living (IADLs) include using things and tools like telephone, money, private or public means of transport, and doing things such as cooking, etc. IADLs are the first impaired in dementia progression. With the cultural growth of the last decades, other activities should be assessed in order to detect the early changes in our patients' behavior, such as employment conduct, hobbies, socializing and involvement in community activities, etc., which can be considered as advanced ADL (AADLs). Lots of validated scales are available: ADL Scale [45], IADL Scale [46], Functional Activities Questionnaire (FAQ) [47], Alzheimer's Disease Cooperative Study (ADCS) ADL Scale [48], Disability Assessment for Dementia (DAD) [49]. The use of such scales is fundamental for the diagnostic work-up and it is highly recommended.

2.6. Evaluation of Behavioral and Psychological Symptoms of Dementia

Another important issue in the diagnostic work-up of dementia is the evaluation of BPSD, which are highly frequent (up to 90%) during the course of the disease [50, 51]. BPSD are usually the cause of faster cognitive impairment and are associated with declining functional abilities and quality of life and with increasing institutionalization. Although their pathogenesis is not yet known, BPSD are often caused by somatic co-morbidities or environmental problems, that trigger anomalous behaviors.

Several scales are available to assess BPSD, and most of them are validated for inter-raters and test-retest reliability. These scales are mostly based on the informants reports and they suffer from the aforementioned biases deriving from emotional and personality traits of the caregivers, who have to bear a highly stressing burden.

The most used scales include the Neuropsychiatric Inventory (NPI) [52], the Cohen-Mansfield Agitation Inventory (CMAI) [53], the Alzheimer's Disease Assessment Scale non-Cog [39], the Ryden Aggression Scale [54], the Behavioral Pathology in Alzheimer's Disease Rating Scale (BEHAVE-AD) [55], and the Behavior Rating Scale for Dementia of the CERAD (CERAD-BRSD) [56]. Among BPSDs, depression plays an important role in managing patients with dementia, and it is very frequent, ranging from 1.5 to 28%, with depressive symptoms up to 87% [57]. Some scales are focused on depression in the elderly, such as the Geriatric Depression Scale (GDS) [58], the Hamilton Depression Scale [59], the Beck Depression Inventory (BDI) [60], but only few of them have been validated for demented people, such as the Cornell Scale for Depression in Dementia (CSDD) [61] and the 15-item Geriatric Depression Scale [62].

The power of these scales is that they are validated in large samples of demented people, giving a quantitative measure of the disturbances, so that it is possible to evaluate the changes in time and the effects of the therapies. However, every scale or questionnaire has its dark side to cope with: being based on the reports from the informants (caregivers or others) they will never be a direct measure of the patients' symptoms.

A psychological assessment of the caregivers should be performed: the somatic and psychological diseases of the caregivers are well known, since there is the necessity of an holistic approach to the disease, taking into account the 'dyad': the caregivers' burden can be evaluated by means of *ad hoc* scales, such as the Caregiver Burden Inventory (CBI) [63], but also through the assessment of personality traits with questionnaires such as the Cattel's 16-Personality Factors [64] which deeply investigates the caregivers' patterns of personality. Moreover, depression, which is the most frequent disturb affecting the caregivers, should be addressed by using specific scales (Hamilton's or Beck's) [59, 60]. Last but not the least, the caregivers' quality of life should be evaluated too, with the appropriate scales, such as the Short Form Health Survey (SF-12) [65].

2.7. Neuroimaging

Our guidelines [8-10] suggest us to carry out a neuroimaging of every patient with dementia, in order to exclude reversible dementias caused by treatable pathologies such as NPH, tumors or chronic subdural hematomas. However, over the age of 60, the indication for at least a neuroimaging exam is not absolute, particularly in case of absence of focal signs or symptoms, seizures, gait impairment, and presence of a slowly progressing course of the cognitive deficit [66]. The computed tomography (CT) can easily exclude any reversible causes of dementia, but it is not able to differentiate between normal ageing and dementia. Easily accessible, being largely available in peripheral hospitals, it is less expensive and fast enough to perform also on severe demented persons, which collaborate very little, as it is very difficult to keep them steady for a long time. Contrast is not indicated; through a specific analysis it is possible to evaluate hippocampal atrophy [67].

Magnetic Resonance Imaging (MRI) is more sensitive, but also more expensive and it needs a good compliance, because the period of acquisition is longer than that for CT, and a demented person may not be able to sustain this effort. Furthermore, a lot of people cannot bear to stay motionless for 20 minutes in a narrow tube because of claustrophobia: sedation is not recommended, because that could be a potential cause of exacerbation of dementia. On these accounts, MRI is only indicated for younger people and under the suspect of vascular infarcts or specific conditions like PSP, MSA, FTD and prion diseases, in which it can give important information with specific radiological patterns [68]. In research setting, MRI is obviously preferable as it allows to measure the exact extent of hippocampal atrophy with new techniques like, for instance, the voxel-based morphometry, and it gives functional patterns with fMRI.

Other functional neuroimaging exams, such as the Single Photon Emission Computed Tomography (SPECT) and the fluorodeoxy-glucose-(FDG-)-

Positron Emission Tomography (PET) are intended to add dynamic information about the cerebral areas involved in neurodegeneration, such as medial temporal (especially hippocampus), basal and lateral temporal lobe, and medial parietal isocortex. SPECT is largely available in Nuclear Medicine Units, usually using ^{99m}Tc-HMPAO or ^{133}Xe, to study regional cerebral blood flow, whose variations depend on brain atrophy; if SPECT shows a defect of perfusion, it can raise diagnostic accuracy of AD to 92%, whereas a negative result lowers the likelihood to 70% [69]. In parametric statistical analysis the SPECT is also useful to tell apart different forms based on the anatomical distribution [70]. Dopaminergic SPECT (DAT Scan) is useful to tell AD and DLB apart [71].

The FDG-PET is more expensive and not immediately available locally, so it is only used in selected cases to differentiate AD from other dementias and in their early stages [72-74]. New ligands for amyloid, like N-methyl-[^{11}C]2-(4′-methylaminophenyl)-6-hydroxybenzothiazole Pittsburgh compound B (PIB), will enable detection of amyloid deposition *in vivo*, also in the preclinical phase of dementia, that is the area of major interest to research in, as it gives a critical opportunity to intervene with disease-modifying therapies. For the time being, PET amyloid imaging is reserved to research settings and indicated as biomarker in Operational Research Criteria (see Tab.6), but in the next future it may become a routine exam for the early diagnosis during the preclinical phase.

2.8. Other Diagnostic Tools

2.8.1. EEG

The Electroencephalography (EEG) is useful in differential diagnosis, although dementia cannot be excluded on the basis of a normal EEG. Creutzfeld-Jacob Disease (CJD), toxic-metabolic disorders and epilepsy may account for EEG abnormalities in subjects with mental deterioration, so it is recommended in atypical presentation of dementia, but it remains an ancillary test [75].

2.8.2. Cerebrospinal Fluid Analysis

Routine Cerebrospinal Fluid (CSF) analysis is necessary whenever inflammatory diseases are suspected, such as vasculitis, multiple sclerosis and so on. In suspected CJD, an increment of 14-3-3 in CSF is expected as a consequence of an acute neuronal loss, as well as high levels of total tau [76].

Reduction in CSF $A\beta_{42}$ is considered an evidence of amyloid-β accumulation in the preclinical phase of AD and, together with increased amyloid PET tracer retention, these are considered the early biomarkers in the Operational Research Criteria (see Tab. 6). In AD, increased total-tau or phospho-tau in CSF are also frequently found, but they are not AD-specific and are considered the biomarkers of a tau-mediated neuronal damage. However, the combined analysis of $A\beta_{42}$ and total- and phospho-tau reach a high sensitivity (85-94%) and specificity (83-100%) in AD versus normal people [77], while the specificity is lower in telling AD apart from other dementias, because of the presence of co-morbid AD pathology [78]. A future challenge in defining CSF biomarkers is to find some absolute data in the concentrations, because there is still too much variance from lab to lab. Besides, these measures are fairly expensive and they are intended to be only used in selected cases (diagnostic doubt) and in research settings.

2.8.3. Genetics

The Apolipoprotein E (APOE) ε4 allele positivity is considered as the major susceptibility gene for late-onset AD [79], but routine genotyping is not recommended. In selected subjects with a family history of several dementia cases or appropriate phenotype (onset at a young age, usually before 60), a screening for genetic risk factors could be undertaken in specialized centers with the appropriate counseling of the patients and family, after having obtained their full consent. The best established early-onset AD-causing mutations are Presenilin 1 (PSEN1), Presenilin 2 (PSEN2), Amyloid Precursor Protein (APP) and Trisomy 21 (Down syndrome). A Huntington's Disease procedure is available for pre-symptomatic testing [80].

Conclusions

A diagnosis of dementia can be carried out following a simple, reasonable framework for all clinicians involved in primary care settings, requiring no excessive economic resources. From the first approach to a complaint of memory loss, a little more time consuming visit should be carried out and assessed, rather than a 'wait-and-see' attitude; this cannot be longer accepted today, since we have new, although symptomatic, treatments available that can improve the quality of life and help to manage this complex disease. Furthermore, an early diagnosis is fundamental and required, as the identification of reversible causes is critical to their treatment, to be able to intervene on co-morbidities with preventions, and, at least, to allow the patients and their families to plan for the future.

In this suggested algorithm (see Figure 1), the diagnosis of dementia is clinical, based on symptoms and signs and exclusion of other causes, and in line with the established criteria (see Tab. 1, 3, 4 and 5).

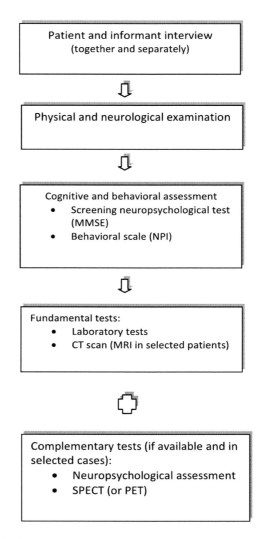

Figure 1. A simple algorithm for clinician diagnosis of dementia.

A pivotal role is played by the interviews with the patients and their informants, in order to collect a detailed history, focused on the everyday life reports about how the cognitive impairment interfere on the patients' activities of daily living. Even if a suspect of dementia can be already delineated on the basis of the anamnesis, a physical and neurological examination should be always carried on in order to look for specific signs.

Afterwards, it is necessary to tell dementia apart from other conditions that could mimic dementia, such as delirium, depression, metabolic conditions or substance abuse.

The following step is to separately consider the various forms of dementia. To that end, a few diagnostic tools may help, economically affordable and available in all the clinical settings. A mental status examination by means of a Mini-mental State Examination or other screening tests is undoubtedly precious, because these tests are flexible for a quantitative as well as for a qualitative use. Sensory impairment (visual deficit or hearing loss) must be carefully considered to prevent the overrating of an impaired performance.

The evaluation of the functional state and psychiatric symptoms (BPSD) with simple scales such as NPI is very informative. At this point, some diagnostic exams are required: firstly, we need to carry out a morphological examination of the brain with a CT scan, better with a quantitative analysis of hippocampal atrophy; secondly, we need to perform a minimal standard battery of lab tests, including blood cell count, electrolytes and calcium, glucose, thyroid stimulating hormone, vitamin B_{12}, folic acid and homocysteine.

Where available, two other diagnostic tools are highly recommended: an extended neuropsychological examination, limited to the mild cognitive impairment and early stage of dementia; a functional investigation, i.e. SPECT (^{99m}Tc-HMPAO or ^{133}Xe) with semi-quantitative assessment. Collected data should be analyzed and compared with the clinical criteria data sets, in order to formulate the hypothesis for our etiological diagnosis. This whole diagnostic framework ideally requires a multidisciplinary approach involving medical specialists (neurologists, psychiatrics, geriatricians, radiologists), psychologists and, desirably, social workers, all acting together to customize interventions to each patient specifically, as we have always a single case, only equal to itself.

What's Next?

Future research is focused on finding more sensitive biomarkers, able to detect the pathologic process which underlies subtle changes in behaviors and variations in daily life activities, and more specific for each different form of dementia. This allows identifying cohorts of persons who will develop dementia, but still in a preclinical phase, when brain damage is not yet consolidated to such extent against which medical treatments are no more effective. The great challenge of our time is to find disease-modifying therapies as, for instance, an intervention that delays the onset of AD by 5 years would result in a 57% reduction in the number of AD patients, and would reduce the projected Medicare costs of AD from 627 to 344 billion dollars [81]. So, PET amyloid imaging and $A\beta_{42}$ on CSF assay are promising biomarkers, but others are needed in order to evaluate larger samples of population without enrolling biases.

For clinical purposes, however, this diagnostic framework seems to be reasonably applicable for the time being, and we here recommend to follow all of its steps.

References

[1]   Bianchetti, A. & Trabucchi, M., (2005). La valutazione clinica del demente. In: Trabucchi M. (Ed.), *Le demenze* (IV ed., 37-101). Torino: UTET.

[2]   Baldereschi, M., Di Carlo, A., Maggi, S. & Inzitari, D. (2005). Le demenze: epidemiologia e fattori di rischio. In: Trabucchi M. (Ed.), *Le demenze* (IV ed., 13-36). Torino: UTET.

[3]   Ritchie, K. & Kildea, D. (1995). Is senile dementia age-related or ageing-related? Evidence from a meta-analysis of dementia prevalence in the oldest old. *Lancet*, 346, 931-934.

[4]   Wirno, A. & Prince, M. (2010). *World Alzheimer Report 2010. The global economic impact of dementia*. London: Alzheimer's Disease International.

[5]   Wimo, A., Jönsson, L., Gustavsson, A., McDaid, D., Ersek, K,, Georges, J., Gulácsi, L., Karpati, K., Kenigsberg, P. & Valtonen, H. (2010). The economic impact of Dementia in Europe in 2008- costs estimated from

the Eurocode project. *International Journal of Geriatric Psychiatry* Pub. online: 28 Oct 2010.

[6]   Blennow, K., de Leon, M.J. & Zetterberg, H. (2006). Alzheimer's disease. *Lancet*, 368, 387-403.

[7]   Chertkow, H., Bergman, H., Schipper, H.M., Gauthier, S., Bouchard, R., Fontaine, S. & Clarfield, A.M. (2001). Assessment of suspected dementia. *The Canadian Journal of Neurological Sciences*, 28, Suppl. 1, S28-S41.

[8]   Knopman, D.S., DeKosky, S.T., Cummings, J.L., Chui, H., Corey-Bloom, J., Relkin, N., Small, G.W., Miller, B. & Stevens, J.C. (2001) Practice parameter: Diagnosis of dementia (an evidence-based review). Report of the Quality Standards Subcommittee of the American Academy of Neurology. *Neurology*, 56, 1143-1153.

[9]   Musicco, M., Caltagirone, C., Sorbi, S., & Bonavita V. (2004) Italian Neurological Society Guidelines for the diagnosis of dementia: I revision. *Neurological Sciences*, 24, 154-182.

[10] Hort, J., O'Brien, J.T., Gainotti, G., Pirttila, T., Popescu, B.O., Rektorova, I., Sorbi, S. & Scheltens, P. (2010). EFNS guidelines for the diagnosis and management of Alzheimer's disease. *European Journal of Neurology*, 17, 1236-1248.

[11] McKhaan, G., Drachman, D., Folstein, M., Katzman, R., Price, D. & Stadlan, E.M. (1984). Clinical diagnosis of Alzheimer's disease: Report of the NINCDS-ADRDA Work Group under the auspices of Department of Health and Human Services Task Force on Alzheimer's Disease. *Neurology*, 34, 939-944.

[12] Spinnler, H. (1985). *Il decadimento demenziale. Inquadramento neurologico e neuropsicologico*. Roma: Il Pensiero Scientifico Editore.

[13] Waldemar, G. (2009). Diagnosing Alzheimer's disease in clinical practice. In: Waldemar, G., & Burns, A. (Eds.) *Alzheimer's Disease* (37-50). New York: Oxford University Press.

[14] Orfei, M. D., Spalletta, G. & Caltagirone, C. (2007). I disturbi della consapevolezza nelle demenze: rilevanza clinica e ipotesi patogenetiche. *Psicogeriatria*, 3, 32-38.

[15] Seiffer, A., Clare, L. & Harvey, R. (2005). The role of personality and coping style in relation to awareness of current functioning in early-stage dementia. *Aging and Mental Health*, 9(6), 535-541.

[16] Clare, L. (2002). Awareness in Dementia: new directions. *Dementia, 1 (3)*, 275-278.

[17] Clare, L. (2004a). The construction of awareness in early-stage Alzheimer's disease: A review of concepts and models. *British Journal of Clinical Psychology, 43,* 155-175.

[18] Clare L. (2004b). Awareness in early-stage Alzheimer's disease: a review of methods and evidence. *British Journal of Clinical Psychology, 43,* 177-196.

[19] Smyth, K. A., Neundorfer, M. M., Koss, E., Geldmacher, D. S., Ogrocki, P. K. & Withehouse, P. J. (2002). Quality of life and deficit identification in dementia. *Dementia, 1(3),* 345-358.

[20] Sacco, L. (2007). La consapevolezza del paziente con demenza. *Traduzione ed adattamento del Questionario di Identificazione dei Deficit.* Congresso Nazionale FERB, 1 giugno 2007, Bergamo.

[21] Vista, M., Picchi, L. & Mazzoni, M. (2010). The caregivers of persons with Alzheimer's disease: The impact of personality traits on own stress perception and in evaluating cognitive and functional impairment of their relatives. In: Jordan, M.E. (Ed.), *Personality Traits Theory, Testing and Influences.* New York: Nova Science Publishers.

[22] Granieri, A. (2002). Teorie, metodi, strumenti e loro interrelazione. In: Granieri A. (Ed.), *I test di personalità: quantità e qualità* (3-24). Torino: UTET.

[23] Seshadri, S., Beiser, A., Selhub, J., Jacques, P.F., Rosenberg, I.H., D'Agostino, R.B., Wilson, P.W.F. & Wolf, P.A. (2002). Plasma homocysteine as a risk factor for dementia and Alzheimer's disease. *The New England Journal of Medicine,* 346, 476-483.

[24] Brodaty, H., Low, L., Gibson, L. & Burns, K. (2006). What is the best dementia screening instrument for General Practitioners to use? *American Journal of Geriatric Psychiatry,* 14 (5), 391-400.

[25] Folstein, M.F., Folstein, S.E. & McHugh, P.R. (1975). 'Mini-mental state'. A practical method for grading the cognitive state of patients for the clinician. *Journal of Psychiatric Research,* 12, 189-198.

[26] Feher, E.P., Mahurin, R.K., Doody, R.S., Cooke, N., Sims, J. & Pirozzolo, F.J. (1992) Estabiling the limits of the Mini-mental State. *Archives of Neurology,* 49 (1), 87-92.

[27] Escobar, J.I., Burnam, A., Karno, M., Forsythe, A., Landsverk, J. & Golding, J.M. (1986) Use of the Mini-mental State Examination (MMSE) in a community population of mixed ethnicity: Cultural and linguistic artifacts. *Journal of Nervous & Mental Disease,* 174 (10): 607-614.

[28] Monsch, A.U., Foldi, N.S., Ermini-Fünfschillin, D.E., Berres, M., Taylor, K.I., Seifritz, E., Stähelin, H.B. & Spiegel, R. (1995). Improving the diagnostic accuracy of the Mini-Mental State Examination, *Acta Neurologica Scandinavica*, 92 (2), 145-150.

[29] Clark, C.M., Sheppard, L, Fillenbaum, G.G., Galasko, D., Morris, J.C., Koss, E., Mohs, R., & Heyman A. (1999). Variability in annual Mini-Mental State Examination score in patients with probable Alzheimer's Disease. *Archives of Neurology*, 56 (7), 857-862.

[30] Dubois, B., Burn, D., Goetz, C., Aarsland, D., Brown, R.G., Broe, G.A., Dickson, D., Duyckaerts, C., Cummings, J., Gauthier, S., Korczyn, A., Lees, A., Levy, R., Litvan, I., Mizuno, Y., McKeith, I.G., Olanow, C.W., Poewe, W., Sampaio, C., Tolosa, E. & Emre, M. (2007). Diagnostic procedures for Parkinson's Disease dementia: Recommendations from the Movement Disorder Society Task Force. *Movement Disorders*, 22, 2314-2324.

[31] Petersen, R.C. (2004). Mild cognitive impairment as a diagnostic entity. *Journal of Internal Medicine,* 256, 183–194.

[32] Petersen, R.C. & Morris, J.C. (2005). Mild Cognitive Impairment as a clinical entity and treatment target. *Archives of Neurology*, 62, 1160-1166.

[33] Albert, M., De Kosky, S., Dickson, D., Dubois, B., Feldman, H., Fox, N., Gamst, A., Holtzman, D., Jagust, W., Petersen, R. & Snyder, P. (2010) *Criteria for Mild Cognitive Impairment due to AD.* Published on line: Alzheimer's Association.

[34] Gainotti, G., Marra, M., Villa, G., Parlato, V. & Chiarotti, F. (1998). Sensitivity and specificity of some neuropsychological markers of Alzheimer Dementia. *Alzheimer Disease and Associated Disorders*, 12 (3), 152-162.

[35] Dubois, B., Feldman, H., Jacova, C., DeKosky, S. T., Barberger-Gateau, P., Cummings, J., Delacourte, A., Galasko, D., Gauthier, S., Jicha, G., Meguro, K., O'Brien, J, Pasquier, F., Robert, P., Rossor, M., Salloway, S., Stern, Y., Visser, P.J., & Scheltens, P. (2007). Research criteria for the diagnosis of Alzheimer's disease: revising the NINCDS-ADRDA criteria. *The Lancet Neurology, 6(8),* 734-746.

[36] Buschke, H., Sliwinki, M.J., Kuslansky, G. & Lipton, R.B. (1997). Diagnosis of early dementia by the Double Memory Test: encoding specificity improves diagnostic sensitivity and specificity. *Neurology*, 48, 989-997.

[37] Copeland, J.R.M., Kelleher, M.J., Kellett, J.M., Gourlay, A.J., Gurland, B.J., Fleiss, J.L., & Sharpe L. (1976). A semi-structured clinical interview for the assessment of diagnosis and mental state in the elderly: The Geriatric Mental State Schedule. 1. Development and reliability. *Psychological Medicine*, 6, 439-449.

[38] Roth, M., Tym, E., Mountjoy, C.Q., Huppert, F.A., Hendrie, H., Verma, S., & Goddard, R. (1986). CAMDEX. A standardised instrument for the diagnosis of mental disorders in the elderly with special reference for the early detection of dementia. *The British Journal of Psychiatry*, 149, 698-709.

[39] Rosen, W.G., Mohs, R., & Davis, K. (1984). A new Rating Scale for Alzheimer's disease. *American Journal of Psychiatry*, 141, 1356-1364.

[40] Brazzelli, M., Capitani, E., Della Sala, S., Spinnler, H. & Zuffi, M. (1994). A neuropsychological instrument adding to the description of patients with suspected cortical dementia: The Milan Overall Dementia Assessment. *Journal of Neurology, Neurosurgery and Psychiatry*, 57, 1510-1517.

[41] Bracco, L., Amaducci, L., Pedone, D., Bino, G., Lazzaro, M.P., Carella, F., D'Antona, R., Gallato, R., & Denes, G. (1990). Italian multicentre study on dementia (SMID): A neuropsychological test battery for assessing Alzheimer's Disease. *Journal of Psychiatric Research*, 24, 213-226.

[42] Caltagirone, C., Gainotti, G., Carlesimo, G.A., Parnetti, L., e il Gruppo per la standardizzazione della batteria per il Deterioramento Mentale (1995). Batteria per la valutazione del Deterioramento Mentale (Parte I): descrizione di uno strumento di diagnosi neuropsicologica. *Archivio di Psicologia, Neurologia e Psichiatria*, 4, 461-470.

[43] Carlesimo, G.A., Caltagirone, C., Gainotti, G, Nocentini, U., e il Gruppo per la standardizzazione della batteria per il Deterioramento Mentale (1995). Batteria per la valutazione del Deterioramento Mentale (Parte II): standardizzazione e affidabilità diagnostica nell'identificazione di pazienti affetti da sindrome demenziale. *Archivio di Psicologia, Neurologia e Psichiatria*, 4, 471-488.

[44] Carlesimo, G.A., Caltagirone, C., Fadda, L., Marfia, G.A., Gainotti, G., e il Gruppo per la standardizzazione della batteria per il Deterioramento Mentale (1995). Batteria per la valutazione del Deterioramento Mentale (Parte III): analisi dei profili qualitativi di compromissione cognitiva. *Archivio di Psicologia, Neurologia e Psichiatria*, 4, 489-502.

[45] Katz, S., Ford, A.B., Moskowitz, R.W., Jackson, B.A., & Jaffe, M.W. (1963). The index of ADL: A standardized measure of biological and psychosocial function. *The Journal of American Medical Association*, 185 (12): 914-919.

[46] Lawton, M.P., & Brody, E.M. (1969) Assessment of older people: Self-maintaining and instrumental activities of daily living. *Gerontologist*, 9,179-186.

[47] Pfeffer, R.I., Kurosaki, T.T., Harrah Jr., C.H., Chance, J.M., & Filos, S. (1982). Measurement of functional activities in older adults in the community. *The Journal of Gerontology*, 37, 323-329.

[48] Galasko, D., Bennett, D., Sano, M., Ernesto, C., Ronald, T., Grundman, M., & Ferris, S. (1997). An inventory to assess activities of daily living for clinical trials in Alzheimer's Disease. *Alzheimer Disease and Associated Disorders*, 11, Suppl 2, S33-S39.

[49] Gelinas, I., Gauthier, L., & McIntyre, M. (1999) Development of a functional measure for persons with Alzheimer's disease: the disability assessment for dementia. *American Journal of Occupational Therapy*, 53, 471-481.

[50] Finkel, S. I. (1996). Behavioural and Psychological Signs and Symptoms of Dementia: Implication for research and treatment. *International Psychogeriatrics*, 8 (suppl.3).

[51] De Vreese, L. P. (2004). *La demenza nell'anziano: dalla diagnosi alla gestione* (47-82). Torino: UTET.

[52] Cummings, J.L., Mega, M., Gray, K., Rosemberg-Thompson, S., Carusi, D.A., & Gornbein, J. (1994). The Neuropsychiatric Inventory: Comprehensive assessment of psychopathology in dementia. *Neurology*, 44, 2308-

[53] Cohen-Mansfield, J., Marx, M.S., & Rosenthal, A.S. (1989). A description of agitation in a nursing home. *Journal of Gerontology: Medical Sciences*, 44 (3), M77-M84.

[54] Ryden, M.B. (1988). Aggressive behavior in persons with dementia who live in the community. *Alzheimer's Disease and Associated Disorders*, 2, 342-355.

[55] Reisenberg, B., Borenstein, J., Salob, S.P., Ferris, S.H., Franssen, E., & Georgotas, A. (1987). Behavioral symptoms in Alzheimer's disease: Phenomenology and treatment. *The Journal of Clinical Psychiatry*, 48 (Suppl.), 9-15.

[56] Tariot, P.N., Mack, J.L., Patterson, M.B., Edland, S.D., Weiner, M.F., Fillenbaum, G., Blazina, L., Teri, L., Rubin, E., & Mortimer, J.A.

(1995). The behavior rating scale for dementia of the consortium to estabilish a registry for Alzheimer-disease. *American Journal of Psychiatry*, 152, 1349-1357.

[57] Wragg, R.E. & Jeste, D.V. (1989) Overview of depression and psychosis in Alzheimer's Disease. *American Journal of Psychiatry*, 146, 577-587.

[58] Yesavage, J.A., Brink, T.L., Rose, T.L., Lum, O., Huang, V., Adey, M., & Leirer, V.O. (1983). Development and validation of a geriatric depression screening scale: A preliminary report. *Journal of Psychiatric Research*, 17, 37-49.

[59] Hamilton, M. (1960). A rating scale for depression. *Journal of Neurology, Neurosurgery and Psychiatry*, 23, 56-62

[60] Beck, A.T., Ward, C.H., Mendelson, M., Mock, J., & Erbaugh, J. (1961). An inventory for measuring depression. *Archives of General Psychiatry*, 4, 561-571.

[61] Alexopoulos, G.S., Abrams, R.C., Young, R.C., & Shamoian, C.A. (1988). Cornell Scale for Depression in Dementia. *Biological Psychiatry*, 23, 271-284.

[62] Sheikh, J.I., & Yesavage, J.A. (1986). Geriatric Depression Scale (GDS): recent evidence and development of a shorter version. *Clinical Gerontologist*, 5, 165-173.

[63] Novak, M. & Guest, C. (1989). Application of a Multidimensional Caregiver Burden Inventory. *Gerontologist, 9,* 169-186.

[64] Cattel, R. B. (1956). *Handbook supplement for Form C of the Sixteen Personality Factor Questionnaire* (16 PF), Champaign, III, Institute for Personality and Ability Testing; trad. it. *16 PF: I sedici fattori della personalità. Forma C.* Firenze: Organizzazioni Speciali, 1978.

[65] Ware, J.E., Kosinski, M., & Keller, S.D. (1996). A 12-item Short-Form Health Survey: construction of scales and preliminary tests of reliability and validity. *Medical Care*, 34, 220-233.

[66] Report of the Quality Standards Subcommittee of the American Academy of Neurology (1994). Practice parameter for diagnosis and evaluation of dementia (Summary statement). *Neurology*, 44, 2203-2206.

[67] Wattjes, M.P., Henneman, W.J., van der Flier, W.M., de Vries, O., Träber, F., Geurts, J.J., Scheltens, P., Vrenken, H., & Barkhof, F. (2009). Diagnostic imaging of patients in a memory clinic: comparison of MR imaging and 64-detector row CT. *Radiology*, 253, 174-183.

[68] Scheltens, P., Fox, N., Barkhof, F., & De Carli, C. (2002) Structural magnetic resonance imaging in the practical assessment of dementia: beyond exclusion. *The Lancet Neurology*, 1, 13-21.

[69] Jagust, W., Thisted, R., Devous, M.D., Van Heertum, R., Mayberg, H., Jobst, K., Smith, A.D., & Borys, N. (2001). SPECT perfusion imaging in the diagnosis of Alzheimer's Disease: a clinical-pathologic study. *Neurology*, 56, 950-956.

[70] Dougall, N.J., Bruggink, S., & Ebmeier, K.P. (2004). Systematic review of the diagnostic accuracy of 99mTc-HMPAO-SPECT in dementia. *American Journal of Geriatric Psychiatry*, 12, 554-570.

[71] McKeith, I., O'Bien, J., Walker, Z., Tatsch, K., Booij, J., Darcourt, J., Padovani, A., Giubbini, R., Bonuccelli, U., Volterrani, D., Holmes, C., Kemp, P., Tabet, N., Meyer, I., Reininger, C., & DLB Study Group (2007) Sensitivity and specificity of dopamine transporter imaging with 123I-FP-CIT SPECT in dementia with Lewy bodies: a phase III, multicentre study. *The Lancet Neurology*, 6, 305-313.

[72] Silverman, D.H., & Alavi, A. (2005). PET imaging in the assessment of normal and imapired cognitive finction. *Radiologic Clinics of North America*, 43, 67-77.

[73] Panegyres, P.K., Rogers, J.M., McCarthy, M., Campbell, A., & Wu, J.S. (2009). Fluorodeoxyglucose-positron emission tomography in the differential diagnosis of early-onset dementia: a prospective, community-based study. *BMC Neurology*, 9, 41-50.

[74] Foster, N.L., Heidebrink, J.L., Clatck, C.M., Jagust, W.J., Arnold, S.E., Barbas, N.R., DeCarli, C.S., Scott Turner, R., Koeppe, R.A., Higdon, R., & Minoshima, S. (2007). FDG-PET improves accuracy in distinguish frontotemporal dementia and Alzheimer's disease. *Brain*, 130 (10), 2616-2635.

[75] Jelic, V., & Kowalski, J. (2009). Evidence-based evaluation of diagnostic accuracy of resting EEG in dementia and mild cognitive impairment. *Clinical EEG & Neuroscience*, 40, 129-142.

[76] Sanchez-Juan, P., Green, A., Ladogana, A., Cuadrado-Corrales, N., Sáanchez-Valle, R., Mitrováa, E., Stoeck, K., Sklaviadis, T., Kulczycki, J., Hess, K., Bodemer, M., Slivarichová, D., Saiz, A., Calero, M., Ingrosso, L., Knighy, R., Janssens, A.C., Van Duijn, C.M., & Zerr, I. (2006). CSF tests in the differential diagnosis of Creutzfeldt-Jakob disease. *Neurology*, 67, 637-643.

[77] Blennow, K., Vanmechelen, E., & Hampel, H. (2001). CSF total tau, Aβ42 and phosphorylated tau protein as biomarkers for Alzheimer's disease. *Molecular Neurobiology*, 24, 87-97.

[78] Tapiola, T., Alafuzoff, I., Herukka, S.K., Parkkinen, L., Hartikainen, P., Soinenen, H., & Pirttilä, T. (2009). CSF beta-amyloid 42 and tau proteins are markers of Alzheimer-type pathology in the brain. *Archives of Neurology*, 66, 382-389.

[79] Brouwers, N., Sleegers, K., & Van Broeckhoven, C. (2008). Molecular genetics of Alzheimer's Disease: an update. *Annals of Medicine*, 40, 562-583.

[80] Tibben, A. (2007). Predictive testing for Huntington's Disease. *Brain Research Bulletin*, 72, 165-171.

[81] Sperling, R., Beckett, L., Bennett, D., Craft, S., Fagan, A., Kaye, J., Montine, T., Park, D., Reiman, E., Siemers, E., Stern, Y., Yaffe, K., Clifford, J., & Aisen, P. (2010). *Criteria for preclinical Alzheimer's Disease.* Published on line: Alzheimer's Association.

[82] World Health Organization (1992). The ICD-10 classification of mental and behavioural disorders. Clinical descriptions and diagnostic guidelines.

[83] McKhann, G., Hyman, B., Jack, C., Kawas, C., Klunk, W., Knopman, D., Koroshetz, W., Manly, J., Mayeux, R., Mohs, R., Morris, J., & Weintraub, S. (2010). *Criteria for AD dementia.* Published on line: Alzheimer's Association.

[84] Alafuzoff, I., Pikkarainen, M., Al Sarraj, S., Arzberger, T., Bell, J., Bodi, I., Bogdanovic, N., Budka, H., Bugiani, O., Ferrer, I., Gelpi, E., Giaccone, G., Graeber, M.B., Hauw, J.J., Kamphorst, W., King, A., Kopp, N., Korkolopoulou, P., Kovacs, G.G., Meyronet, D., Parchi, P., Patsouris, E., Preusser, M., Ravid, R., Roggendorf, W., Seilhean, D., Streichenberger, N., Thal, D.R., & Kretzschmar, H. (2006). Interlaboratory comparison of assessments of Alzheimer disease-related lesions: a study of the BrainNet Europe Consortium. *Journal of Neuropathology and Experimental Neurology*, 65, 740–757.

[85] Braak, H., & Braak, E. (1991) Neuropathological stageing of Alzheimer-related changes. *Acta Neuropathologica*, 82, 239–259.

[86] Consensus recommendations for the postmortem diagnosis of Alzheimer's disease. The National Institute on Aging, Reagan Institute Working Group on Diagnostic Criteria for the Neuropathological Assessment of Alzheimer's Disease. (1997). *Neurobiology of Aging,* 18, S1–S2.

[87] Mirra, S.S., Heyman, A., McKeel, D., Sumi, S.M., Crain, B.J., Brownlee, L.M., Vogel, F.S., Hughes, J.P., van Belle, G., & Berg, L. (1991) The Consortium to Establish a Registry for Alzheimer's Disease (CERAD). Part II. Standardization of the neuropathologic assessment of Alzheimer's disease. *Neurology*, 41, 479–486.

[88] McKeith, I.G., Galasko, D., Kosaka, K., Perry, E.K., Dickson, D.W., Hansen, L.A., Salmon, D.P., Lowe, J., Mirra, S.S., Byrne, E.J., Lennox, G., Quinn, N.P., Edwardson, J.A., Ince, P.G., Bergeron, C., Burns, A., Miller, B.L., Lovestone, S., Collerton, D., Jansen, E.N.H., Ballard, C., de Vos, R.A.I., Wilcock, G.K., Jellinger, K.A., & Perry, R.H. (1996). Consensus Guidelines for the clinical and pathologic diagnosis of dementia with Lewy bodies (DLB): Report of the consortium on DLB international workshop. *Neurology*, 47, 1113-1124.

[89] McKeith, I.G., Perry, E.K., & Perry R.H. (1999). Report of the second dementia with Lewy body international workshop. Diagnosis and treatment. *Neurology*, 53, 902-905.

[90] McKeith, I.G., Dickson, D.W., Lowe, J., Emre, M., O'Brien, J.T., Feldman, H., Cummings, J., Duda, J.E., Lippa, C., Perry, E.K., Aarsland, D., Arai, H., Ballard, C.G., Boeve, B., Burn, D.J., Costa, D., Del Ser, T., Dubois, B., Galasko, D., Gauthier, S., Goetz, C.G., Gomez-Tortosa, E., Halliday, G., Hansen, L.A., Hardy, J., Iwatsubo, T., Kalaria, R.N., Kaufer, D., Kenny, R.A., Korczyn, A., Kosaka, K., Lee, V.M.-Y., Lees, A., Litvan, I., Londos, E., Lopez, O.L., Minoshima, S., Mizuno, Y., Molina, J.A., Mukaetova-Ladinska, E.B., Paquier, F., Perry, R.H., Schulz, J.B., Trojanowski, J.Q., & Yamada, M. (2005). Diagnosis and management of dementia with Lewy bodies. Third report of the DLB consortium. *Neurology*, 65, 1863-1872.

[91] Brun, A., Englund, B., Gustafson, L., Passant, U., Mann, D.M.A., Neary, D., & Snowden, J.S. (1994). Clinical and neuropathological criteria for frontotemporal dementia. *Journal of Neurology, Neurosurgery and Psychiatry*, 57, 416-418.

[92] Neary, D., Snowden, J.S., Gustafson, L., Passant, U., Stuss, D., Black, S, Freedman, M., Kertesz, A., Robert, P.H., Albert, M., Boone, K., Miller, B.L., Cummings, J., & Benson, D.F. (1998). Frontotemporal lobar degeneration: a consensus on clinical diagnostic criteria. *Neurology*, 51, 1546-1554.

[93] McKhann, G.M., Albert, N.S., Grossman, M., Miller, B., Dickson, D., & Trojanowski, J.Q. (2001). Clinical and pathological diagnosis of

frontotemporal dementia: report of the Work Group on Frontotemporal Dementia and Pick's Disease. *Archives of Neurology*, 58, 1803-1809.

[94] Cairns, N.J., Bigio, E.H., Mackenzie, I.R.A., Neumann, M., Lee, V. M.-Y., Hatanpaa, K.J., White III, C.L., Schneider, J.A., Tenenholtz Grinberg, L, Halliday, G., Duyckaerts, C., & Lowe, J.S. (2007). Neuropathologic diagnostic and nosologic criteria for frontotemporal lobar degeneration: consensus of the Consortium for Frontotemporal Lobar Degeneration. *Acta Neuropathologica*, 114 (1), 5-22.

[95] Braak, H., Ghebremedhin, E., Rub, U., Bratzke, H., & Del Tredici, K. (2004) Stages in the development of Parkinson's disease-related pathology. *Cell & Tissue Research*, 318, 121–134.

[96] Emre, M., Aarsland, D., Brown, R., Burn, D.J., Duyckaerts, C., Mizuno, Y., Broe, G.A., Cummings, J., Dickson, D.W., Gauthier, S., Goldman, J., Goetz, C., Korczyn, A., Lees, A., Levy, R., Litvan, I., Mckeith, I., Olanow, W., Poewe, W., Quinn, N., Sampaio, C., Tolosa, E., & Dubois, B. (2007). Clinical diagnostic criteria for dementia associated with Parkinson's Disease. *Movement Disorders*, 22, 1689-1707.

[97] Hauw, J.J., Daniel, S.E., Dickson, D., Horoupian, D.S., Jellinger, K., Lantos, P.L., McKee, A., Tabaton, M., & Litvan, I. (1994). Preliminary NINDS neuropathologic criteria for Steele-Richardson-Olszewski syndrome (progressive supranuclear palsy). *Neurology*, 44, 2015–2019.

[98] Litvan, I., Agid, Y., Calne, D., Campbell, G., Dubois, B., Duvoisin, R.C., Goetz, C.G., Golbe, L.I., Grafman, J., Growdon, J.H., Hallett, M., Jankovic, J., Quinn, N.P., Tolosa, E., & Zee, D.S. (1996). Clinical research criteria for the diagnosis of progressive supranuclear plasy (Steele-Richardson-Olszewski syndrome): report of the NINDS-SPSP International workshop. *Neurology*, 47, 1-9.

[99] Boeve, B.F., Maraganore, D.M., Parisi, J.E., Ahlskog, J.E., Graff-Radford, N., Caselli, R.J., Dickson, D.W., Kokmen, E., & Petersen, R.C. (1999) Pathologic heterogeneity in clinically diagnosed corticobasal degeneration. *Neurology*; 53(4), 795-800.

[100] Riley, D., & Lang, A. (2000). Corticobasal degeneration. *Advanced in Neurology*, 82, 29-34.

[101] Dickson, D.W., Bergeron, C., Chin, S.S., Duyckaerts, C., Horoupian, D., Iked, K., Jellinger, K., Lantos, P.L., Lippa, C.F., Mirra, S.S., Tabaton, M., Vonsattel, J.P., Wakabayashi, K., & Litvan, I. (2002). Office of Rare Disease Neuropathologic Criteria for Corticobasal Degeneration. *Journal of Neuropathology & Experimental Neurology*, 61 (11), 935-946.

[102] American Psychiatric Association (1994). *DSM-IV. Diagnostic and Statistic Manual of Mental Disorders*, 4th ed. Washington, DC

[103] Callahan, C.M., Unverzagt, F.W., Hui, S.L., Perkins, A.J., & Hendrie, H.C. (2002). Six-item screener to identify cognitive impairment amomg potential subjects for clinical research. *Medical Care*, 40, 771-781.

[104] Lee, H., Swanwick, G.R., Coen, R.F., & Lawlor, B.A. (1996). Use of the clock drawing task in the diagnosis of mild and very mild Alzheimer's disease. *International Psychogeriatric*, 8, 469-476.

[105] Cullum, C.M., Thompson, L.L., & Smernoff, E.N. (1993). Three-word recall as a measure of memory. *Journal of Clinical and Experimental Neuropsychology*, 15, 321-329.

[106] Borson, S. (2000). The mini-cog: a cognitive "vital signs" measure for dementia screening in multilingual elderly. *International Journal of Geriatric and Psychiatry*, 15 (11), 1021-.

[107] Buschke, H., Kuslanski, G., Katz, M., Stewart, W.F., Sliwinski, M.J., Eckholdt, H.M., & Lipton, R.B. (1999). Screening for dementia with the Memory Impairment Screen. *Neurology*, 52, 231-.

[108] Mendiondo, M.S., Ashford, J.W., Kryscio, R.J., & Schmitt, F.A. (2003). Designing a brief Alzheimer screen (BAS). *Journal of Alzheimer's Disease*, 5, 391-398.

[109] Galvin, J.E., Roe, C.M., Powlishta, K.K., Coats, M.A., Muich, S.J., Grant, E., Miller, J.P., Storandt, M, & Morris, J.C. (2005) The AD8: A brief informant interview to detect dementia. *Neurology*, 65, 559-564.

[110] Brodaty, H., Pond, D., Kemp, N.M., Luscombe, G., Harding, L., Berman, K., & Huppert, F.A. (2002). The GPCOG: a new screening test for dementia designed for general practice. *Journal of the American Geriatrics Society*, 50, 530-534.

[111] Katzman, R., Brown, T., Fuld, P., Peck, A., Schechter, R., & Schimmel, H. (1983) Validation of a short orientation-memory concentration test of cognitive impairment. *American Journal of Psychiatry*, 140, 734-739.

[112] Brandt, J., & Benedict, R.H.B. (2001). *Hopkins Verbal Learning Test— Revised. Professional manual.* Lutz, FL: Psychological Assessment Resources, Inc.

[113] Hodkinson, H.M. (1972) Evaluation of a mental test score for assessment of mental impairment in the elderly. *Age and Ageing*, 1, 233-238.

[114] Jorm, A.F. (2004). The Informant Questionnaire on Cognitive Decline in the Elderly (IQCODE): A review. *International Psychogeriatrics*, 16, 1-19.

[115] Solomon, P.R., Hirshoff, A., Kelly, B., Relin, M., DeVeaux, R.D., & Pendelbury, W.W. (1998). A 7 minute neurocognitive screening battery highly sensitive to Alzheimer's disease. *Archives of Neurology*, 55, 349-355.

[116] Kokmen, E., Naessens, J.M., & Offord, K.P. (1987). A short test of mental status: description and preliminary results. *Mayo Cinic Proceedings*, 62, 281-288.

[117] Inouye, S.K., Robison, J.T., Froelich, T.E., & Richardson, E.D. (1998). The time and change test: a simple screening test for dementia. *Journals of Gerontology Series A: Biological Sciences and Medical Sciences*, 53, M281-M286.

[118] Jones, B.N., Teng, E.L., Folstein, M.F., & Harrison, K.S.. (1993). A new bedside test of cognition for patients with HIV infection. *Annals of Internal Medicine*, 119, 1001-1004.

[119] Brandt, J., Spencer, M., & Folstein, M. (1988). The telephone interview for cognitive status. *Neuropsychiatry, Neuropsychology and Behavioural Neurology*, 1, 111–117.

[120] Mioshi, E., Dawson, K., Mitchell, J., Arnold, R., & Hodges, J.R. (2006). The Addenbrooke's Cognitive Examination Revised (ACE-R): a brief cognitive test battery for dementia screening. *International Journal of Geriatrics Psychiatry*, 21, 1078-1085.

[121] Nasreddine, Z.S., Phillips, N.A., Bédirian, V., Charbonneau, S., Whitehead, V., Collin, I., Cummings, J.L., & Chertkow, H. (2005). The Montreal Cognitive Assessment, MoCA: a brief screening tool for mild cognitive impairment. *Journal of the American Geriatrics Society*, 53, 695-699.

[122] Rascovsky, K., Salmon, D.P., Hansen, L.A., & Galsko, D. (2008). Distinct cognitive profiles and rates of decline on the Mattis Dementia Rating Svale in autopsy-confirmed frontotemporal dementia and Alzheimer's disease. *Journal of the International Neuropsychological Society*, 14, 373-383.

[123] Chandler, M.J., Lacritz, L.H., Hynan, L.S., Barnard, H.D., Allen, G., Deschner, M., Weirner, M.F., & Cullum, C.M. (2005). A total score for the CERAD neuropsychological battery. *Neurology*, 65, 102-106.

[124] Kiernan, R.J., Mueller, J., Langston, J.W., & Van Dyke, C. (1987). The Neurobehavioral Cognitive Status Examination: A brief but differentiated approach to cognitive assessment. *Annals of Internal Medicine*, 107, 481-485.

[125] Robert, P.H., Schuck, S., Dubois, B., Oilé, J.P., Lépine, J.P., Gallarda, T., Goni, S., & Troy, S. (2003), Screening for Alzheimer's disease with the short cognitive evaluation battery. *Dementia and Geriatrics Cognitive Disorders*, 15, 92-98.

[126] Storey, J.E., Rowland, J.T., Basic, D., Conforti, D.A., & Dickson, H.G. (2004). The Rowland Universal Assessment Scale (RUDAS): a multicultural cognitive assessment scale. *International Psychogeriatrics*, 16, 13-31.

[127] Belle, S.H., Mendelsohn, A.B., Seaberg, E.C., & Ratcliff, G. (2000). A brief cognitive screening battery for dementia in the community. *Neuroepidemiology*, 19, 43-50.

[128] Pfeffer, R.I., Kurosaki, T.T., Harrah, C.H. jr, Chance, J.M., & Filos, S. (1982). Measurement of functional activities in older adults in the community. *The Journal of Gerontology*, 37, 323-329.

[129] Bland, R.C., & Newman, S.C. (2001). Mild dementia or cognitive impairment: the Modified Mini-Mental State Examination (3MS) as a screen for dementia. *Canadian Journal of Psychiatry*, 46,506-510.

[130] Drachman, D.A., Swearer, J.M., Kane, K., Osgood, D., O'Toole, C., & Moonis, M. (1996). The Cognitive Assessment Screening Test (CAST) for dementia. *Journal of Geriatric, Psychiatry and Neurology*, 9, 200-208.

[131] Roth, M., Huppert, F., & Tym, E. (1988). *The Cambridge Examination for Mental Disorders of the Elderly*. Cambridge: Cambridge University Press.

[132] Hall, K.S., Gao, S., Emsley, C.L., Oqunnivi, A.O., Morgan, O., & Hendrie, H.C. (2000) Community screening interview for dementia (CSI 'D'): performance in five disparate study sites. *International Journal of Geriatrics Psychiatry,* 15, 521-531.

[133] Silverman, J.M., Breitner, J.C., Mohs, R.C., & Davis, K.L. (1986) Reliability of the family history method in genetic studies of Alzheimer's Disease and related disorders. *American Journal of Psychiatry*, 143, 1279-1282.

In: Alzheimer's Diagnosis   ISBN: 978-1-61209-846-3
Editor: Charles E. Ronson, pp. 175-225   ©2011 Nova Science Publishers, Inc.

Chapter VIII

The Role of Neuroimaging in the Early Diagnosis of Alzheimer's Disease

*Valentina Garibotto** *and Daniela Perani*

IRCCS San Raffaele Scientific Institute, Milano, Italy;
Vita-Salute San Raffaele University, Milano, Italy

Abstract

The demographics of aging suggest a great need for an early diagnosis of dementia and for the development of preventive strategies.

Neurodegeneration in Alzheimer's disease (AD) is estimated to start even 20–30 years before clinical onset, and the identification of biological markers for pre-clinical and early diagnosis is the principal aim of research studies in the field.

It is still difficult to make diagnosis in the early disease stages. At the beginning the patient might have a deficit limited to memory or to another single cognitive domain, without any disorder of instrumental and daily activities. The cognitive impairment then

* Correspondence concerning this article should be addressed to: Valentina Garibotto, garibotto.valentina@hsr.it.

might proceed to a degree that allows the diagnosis of dementia. The transitional state between normal ageing and mild dementia has been recently indicated by the term Mild Cognitive Impairment (MCI).

In the last few years, a wide range of studies addressed this topic. Clinically, within the group of MCI subjects, two separate subgroups have been described, those rapidly converting to AD (MCI converters), in whom MCI represents the early stage of an ongoing AD-related process, and those who remain stable (MCI non-converters), in whom the isolated cognitive deficits represent a different condition without an increased risk to develop dementia at short follow-up.

In this line, reliable markers for early AD detection could be useful both for prognosis, and for identifying a potential target for therapeutic intervention, since treatments are emerging which rather than reversing structural damage are likely to slow or halt the disease process.

While currently no routine diagnostic test confirms AD presence, functional neuroimaging techniques represent an important tool in biological neurology. The challenge for neuroimaging methods is to achieve high specificity and sensitivity in early disease stages and at single subject level. Functional imaging, in particular, has the potential to detect very early brain dysfunction even before clear-cut neuropsychological deficits emerge. Predicting progression to AD in cases of MCI and supporting diagnosis and differential diagnosis of dementia are the outmost important goals.

The implications are the identification of minimally symptom-matic patients that could benefit from treatment strategies, as well as the monitoring of treatment response and the therapeutic decal-eration of the disease.

This chapter highlights recent cross-sectional and longitudinal neuroimaging studies in the attempt to put into perspective their value in diagnosing AD-like changes, particularly at an early stage, providing diagnostic and prognostic specificity.

There is now considerable evidence supporting that early diagnosis is feasible through a multimodal approach, including also a combination of multiple imaging modalities.

1. Introduction

Age is a major risk factor for neurodegenerative diseases in general and particularly for dementia. Dementia represents a major burden for many countries where life expectancy and therefore proportion of aged people is growing: the incidence of dementia is expected to double during the next 20 years (Katzman and Fox, 1999). Alzheimer's disease (AD) is the most common cause of dementia in all age groups, and account for the 50 to 75% of all cases (Kawas, 2003).

This prospect has led to a considerable effort to unravel the pathophysiologic mechanisms of AD and for the development of effective treatments against this devastating disease. Over the last years, significant progress in the understanding of some of the pathophysiologic mechanisms involved in AD has been made (Dickson, 2003).

The impairment of cognitive functions in dementia is the consequence of a severe loss of functioning synapses and neurons in the brain, in particular in limbic and neocortical association areas.

Histopathologically, AD is characterized by the accumulation of senile plaques and neurofibrillary tangles. Whereas the senile plaques consist mainly of β-amyloid peptides, the fibrillary tangles consist of abnormal hyperphosphorylated insoluble forms of the τ-protein. Not much is known about how these two lesions influence each other, e.g., if the hyper-phosphorylation of τ-proteins is triggered by the accumulation of β-amyloid oligomers (amyloid cascade hypothesis) or if a defect in the τ-protein leads to an accumulation of β-amyloid (τ and tangle hypothesis) (Morris and Mucke, 2006). Both lesions can exert direct and indirect neurotoxic effects and promote neuronal death by inducing oxidative stress and inflammation (DeKosky, 2003; Praticò et al., 2002).

The neurofibrillary pathology in AD develops at first in the transentorhinal and entorhinal regions, then spreads into the hippocampus, the limbic system, and finally to neocortical regions (Braak and Braak, 1991).

While the pathway of the neurofibrillary tangles is very precise, the amyloid deposition seems to be more heterogeneous and random, starting first in neocortical regions before it affects allocortical regions and diencephalic structures (Dickson, 2003; Götz et al., 2004; Mudher and Lovestone, 2002; Soto, 2003; Taylor et al., 2002). The analysis of the amino acid sequence of β-amyloid allowed for the identification of the gene encoding its precursor, the β-amyloid precursor protein (APP) on chromosome 21, and thus for the identification of the first series of mutations associated with increased amyloid production and AD. However, such mutations account only for a small percentage of AD cases. The majority of AD patients suffer from sporadic AD for which several risk factors in addition to age have been proposed and are currently being explored, e.g., apolipoprotein E4 (ApoE4), hyperhomocysteinemia, hyperlipidemia, and disturbances of the neuronal insulin signal transduction pathway (Bertram and Tanzi, 2004).

Effective treatment is eagerly awaited. Some drugs that have a moderate symptomatic effect, such as the cholinesterase inhibitors, are already available and some studies indicate that they are able to postpone progression by several months (Winblad et al., 2006). Although the etiology of AD is still not completely clear, the increasing knowledge about some of the most important pathomechanisms in AD allows now for the first time to develop drugs aimed at modifying particular aspects of the AD disease process, e.g., anti-inflammatory drugs, statins, antioxidants, acetylcholinesterase inhibitors, γ and β secretase inhibitors, β sheet disruptors, immunotherapy, neuro-protective agents, or neuroregenerative treatments (see (Dickson, 2003; Irizarry and Hyman, 2001; Knopman, 2006; Mayeux and Sano, 1999; Mudher and Lovestone, 2002) for more detailed reviews). Some of these compounds showed promising results in animal models and are currently being tested in clinical treatment trials in AD patients. In any case, an efficient treatment needs to be installed before a large number of synapses and neurons have been damaged irreversibly, and therefore early markers of disease have a central role.

2. Markers of Early Diagnosis of AD

The rapid scientific progresses on AD biology and the forthcoming clinical trials with disease modifying therapies have heightened the urgency to develop sensitive and reliable biological markers to diagnose and monitor AD activity during life.

The definite diagnosis of AD requires not only the presence of severe cognitive deficits but also autopsy confirmation of the presence of the typical AD histopathologic changes in the brain (Dubois et al., 2007).

In a living person, the diagnosis of possible or probable AD is based on the presence of cognitive deficits in two or more domains severe enough to interfere with normal daily functioning. Although the sensitivity of standardized clinical criteria like the Diagnostic and Statistical Manual of Mental Disorders (DSM-IV), and the National Institute of Neurological, Communicative Disorders, and Stroke-AD and Related Disorders Association (NINCDS-ADRDA) definitions is rather high, i.e., 81% for probable AD and 93% for possible AD, their specificity is lower, i.e., 70% for probable AD and

48% for possible AD (Knopman et al., 2001). Overall, DSM-IV and NINCDS–ADRDA criteria, validated against neuropathological gold standards, reach a diagnostic accuracy ranging from 65–96%, and a specificity against other dementias of only 23–88% (Dubois et al., 2007).

This low specificity likely reflects the fact that AD shares many clinical features with other forms of dementia, and must be addressed through both revised AD and accurate non-AD dementia diagnostic criteria.

Although clinical criteria for the diagnosis of AD in the early to middle stages of the disease may not be perfect, its diagnosis in the very early or asymptomatic stage is an even greater challenge. There is now increasing evidence that the molecular pathomechanisms of AD become active several years before neurons start dying and cognitive deficits manifest (DeKosky and Marek, 2003).

During this stage, an effective treatment of AD would have the greatest impact because the cognitive function could be preserved at the highest level possible. Consequently, there has been considerable interest in recent years to characterize the earliest clinical signs of the degenerative process that is likely to evolve to AD. This effort led to the development of the concept of Mild Cognitive Impairment (MCI), which represents the transitional zone between normal aging and AD. Subjects with MCI are not demented but have significant but very mild deficits in one or more cognitive domains and have an increased risk of dementia (Petersen et al., 2001; Winblad et al., 2004). Depending on which cognitive domains are impaired, different subtypes of MCI can be distinguished. The subtype most relevant for AD is amnestic MCI, which is defined by the presence of subjective memory problems and an objective memory impairment relative to the appropriate reference group, but otherwise normal general cognitive functions and largely preserved activities of daily living (Petersen, 2004).

The annual conversion rate of amnestic MCI to AD is about 15% (range, 6% to 25%) per year, which is considerably higher than the conversion rate of 1% to 2% per year observed for age-matched non-MCI subjects (Gauthier et al., 2006). Histopathologic studies have found that MCI subjects, as a group, usually have intermediate levels of AD pathology compared with healthy controls and subjects with probable or possible AD (Bennett et al., 2005). However, whereas the concept of MCI is very useful to identify a group of subjects with a high risk of conversion to AD, it includes also a non-negligible number of subjects whose disease never converts to AD, or in whom a different form of dementia will develop and thus with different prognosis and perhaps no benefit from AD-specific treatment. Therefore, additional measures that might help to more reliably distinguish between these two MCI categories are needed.

Because of the limitations of clinical and neuropsychological measures for diagnosis and monitoring of treatment effects, there has been considerable effort recently to identify additional biomarkers that might provide complementary information. Diagnostic markers will be also required to support treatment of patients at risk for AD. Of equal significance are markers with the capacity to monitor the underlying biological burden of disease in terms of extent and intensity. These markers will eventually prove to be important surrogate outcome measures in clinical trials supplementing existing clinical data.

Potential biomarkers include blood and CSF measurements of protein concentrations, gene screening, and also, importantly, neuroimaging.

The characteristics of an ideal diagnostic biomarker for AD have been summarized as follows (The Ronald and Nancy Reagan Research Institute of the Alzheimer's Association and, 1998):

1. The biomarker should detect a fundamental feature of the pathophysiologic processes active in AD.
2. The biomarker should be validated in neuropathologically confirmed AD cases.
3. The biomarker has to be precise, i.e., able to detect AD early in its course and distinguish it from other dementias.
4. The measurement of the biomarker has to be reliable, minimally invasive, simple to perform, and inexpensive.

3. Neuroimaging as Biomarker in AD

Traditionally, imaging, and in particular structural imaging, has been used to exclude potentially reversible brain processes mimicking the clinical symptoms of AD, e.g., brain tumours or epidural haematomas.

Recently, however, the potential of neuroimaging, not only to improve the accuracy of the clinical diagnosis of AD, but also to monitor disease progression and treatment effects, has been increasingly recognized.

Imaging might be particularly helpful in providing a marker for disease in early and preclinical phases of AD. Attributes of neuroimaging that make it even superior to neuropsychological tests in AD include increased diagnostic accuracy, freedom from ethnic/cultural bias for interpretation, independence from level or quality of education, and rater-independent objective measures of brain function (Zamrini et al., 2004).

Power analyses showed that neuroimaging as outcome markers in treatment trials would allow for substantially smaller patient populations and shorter observation times than cognitive or clinical outcome measures currently do. Alexander and colleagues calculated that 36 patients in each group (placebo or drug group) would be needed to detect a 33% treatment response with 80% power in a 1-year PET study (Alexander et al., 2002). Jack and colleagues determined that 69 patients in each group would be necessary to detect a 25% treatment effect with 90% power in a 1-year MRI study (Jack et al., 2004). In comparison, at least 1277 patients in each arm would be necessary to detect a 25% treatment effect with 90% power with a cognitive outcome measure (Alexander et al., 2002; Fox et al., 2000; Jack et al., 2004; Reiman et al., 2001).

Recent reviews discuss in detail the increasingly important role played by neuroimaging in clinical trials (Cummings et al., 2007; Thal et al., 2006).

There are two main categories of neuroimaging:

1. structural imaging, which includes Computer-assisted Tomography (CT) and Magnetic Resonance Imaging (MRI)
2. functional imaging, which includes emission tomography techniques, such as Single Photon Emission Computed Tomography (SPECT) and Positron Emission Tomography (PET), and functional Magnetic Resonance Imaging (fMRI).

Functional neuroimaging studies, in particular, are playing a growingly important role in neuropathological and neuropsychological research of dementia, including innovative aspects, such as cognitive activation and *in vivo* studies of neurotransmitter function.

Functional brain imaging offers potential insights into all of the main pathological features of AD – neuronal loss, tangle deposition, cholinergic depletion and amyloid plaques, and also allows measuring the neuro-physiological correlates of disease-related changes in the brain. We will briefly recapitulate the main findings obtained with structural neuroimaging, to then focus on functional neuroimaging, which has a greater potential, mainly in early disease phase.

3.1. Structural MRI

Both CT and MRI have been used for providing structural information on tissue atrophy in AD. However, MRI has several advantages compared with CT: higher resolution, optimal angulation of the imaging plane, excellent grey–white matter discrimination, and identification of additional vascular lesions, particular small lacunes and white matter lesions. All of these factors probably contribute to the higher sensitivity and specificity of MRI (sensitivity, 80% to 94%; specificity, 60% to 100%) for the diagnosis of AD compared with CT (sensitivity, 63% to 88%; specificity, 81%) (Frisoni, 2001).

Several studies have found a good correlation between degree of atrophy on structural imaging and histopathologically confirmed neuron loss and AD pathology (Jack et al., 2002; Silbert et al., 2003; de Leon et al., 2007) and between progression of cognitive impairment and atrophy rate (Fox et al., 1999; Jack et al., 2004).

Changes in structural images are assessed by either qualitative visual assessment or by quantitative volumetric measurements of the entire brain or a structure of interest, i.e., medial temporal lobe or hippocampus. Visual assessments use a qualitative score system, with the advantage of being fast, but the disadvantage of being very subjective and highly dependent on the rater experience. Quantitative volumetric measurements use either a single measure, e.g., radial width of the temporal horn (Chetelat and Baron, 2003), or manual outline the whole structure of interest, e.g., entorhinal cortex. However, particularly the latter method requires some expertise and is time consuming. Therefore, semiautomated and automated computer-based methods, e.g., tissue segmentation, voxel-based morphometry (VBM), or tensor-based morphometry, which in addition have the advantage to assess the entire brain and are not restricted to a single region of interest, are being used increasingly for volumetric studies.

In particular, VBM is an extensively validated approach that allowed the identification of grey and white matter atrophy patterns specific for neurodegenerative processes not only in AD (Borroni et al., 2007; Borroni et al., 2008 ; Whitwell and Jack, 2005).

Mirroring the progression of the tangle pathology, atrophic changes detected by structural imaging affect primarily the entorhinal cortex and hippocampus in the stage of MCI, progress to temporal and parietal lobes in AD, and finally involve also the frontal lobes in late stages of AD (Chetelat and Baron, 2003; Du et al., 2004; Jack et al., 2004; Karas et al., 2004; de Leon et al., 2007; deToledo-Morrell et al., 2004).

Unfortunately, neuron loss and atrophy are not specific for AD but are also found in normal aging or other neurodegenerative diseases.

However, large cross-sectional and longitudinal studies have shown that there are substantial qualitative and quantitative differences in pattern and rate of atrophy in aging and AD, which allow a differentiation of these two processes.

For example, in normal aging, rates of global atrophy typically increase from 0.2% per year at age 30 to 50 to 0.3% to 0.5% per year at age 70 to 80 and affect frontal and parietal grey matter more than occipital and temporal grey matter, whereas changes in white matter are more diffuse (Resnick et al., 2003). In AD, brain atrophy rates are significantly higher, i.e., up to 2% to 3 % per year (Fox and Schott, 2004; Gunter et al., 2003) and so are atrophy rates of hippocampus (controls, 1.0% to 1.2% per year; AD, 3.0% to 5.9% per year) and in entorhinal cortex (controls, 1.4% to 2.9% per year; AD, 7.1% to 8.4% per year), all structures known to be affected early in AD (Du et al., 2004; Jack et al., 2004).

MCI patients have significant hippocampal atrophy when compared to aged normal controls. When comparing patients with probable AD to MCI subjects, hippocampal region atrophy significantly extends to the neighboring temporal association neocortex (Chetelat and Baron, 2003). Comparing the initial MRI data of at-risk subjects who convert to AD at follow-up to those of non-converters suggests that a reduced association temporal neocortex volume combined with hippocampal or anterior cingulate cortex atrophy may be the best predictor of progression to AD (Dickerson et al., 2001; Visser et al., 1999). A recent longitudinal study has specifically addressed this issue, observing a significantly greater gray matter loss in converters relative to non-converters in the hippocampal area, inferior and middle temporal gyrus, posterior cingulate, and precuneus (Boxer et al., 2006).

Although there is some overlap between the brain regions with the most pronounced atrophy in AD and atrophied brain in other types of dementia, degree of atrophy and pattern of involved brain areas seem to be useful for supporting a differentiation between various forms of dementia, describing patterns specific for the various nosologic entities, e.g., Lewy Body Dementia (LBD), Parkinson's disease with dementia (PDD), Fronto-Temporal Lobar Degeneration (FTLD) (Ballmaier et al., 2004; Borroni et al., 2007; Borroni et al., 2008; Burton et al., 2004; Chételat et al., 2005; Rabinovici et al., 2007; Tam et al., 2005). An example of the results provided by such an approach is shown in Figure 1, showing the pattern of grey matter atrophy in the two major variants of Frontotemporal Dementia (FTD), frontal and temporal variants, respectively. VBM comparison with healthy controls is able to reveal a selective atrophy, involving dorsolateral frontal cortex, anterior cingulate cortex, insula, superior temporal gyrus in patients with the frontal variant of FTD, and left middle and inferior temporal gyrus and superior frontal and orbitofrontal gyrus in patients with the temporal variant of FTD (Borroni et al., 2007).

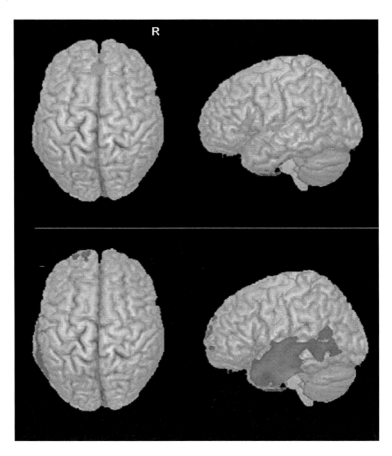

Figure 1. Results of a voxel based morphometry analysis of grey matter atrophy in patients with Frontotemporal Dementia (FTD), showing a different pattern of atrophy in the two major clinical variants of FTD: frontal variant (upper panel) and temporal variant (lower panel). See text for details.

All the studies previously mentioned are based on the comparison of groups of subjects, but an ideal biomarker should be able to provide useful information investigating single subjects.

In this direction, two analysis methods for volumetric MRI data are currently tested and used, with very promising results.

Tensor-based morphometry (TBM) evaluates longitudinal changes in single subjects, to identify regions of faster progression of grey matter atrophy, as compared to controls (Kipps et al., 2005; Leow et al., 2007). A few recent papers have demonstrated its usefulness describing differential patterns of progression in dementias (Brambati et al., in press; Brambati et al., 2007; Thompson et al., 2007).

A cortical thickness measurement, obtained with a specific surface reconstruction process, has been used to detect the characteristic patterns of cortical thinning in AD, MCI, and other types of dementia, and to test the relationship between cortical thickness and cognitive impairment (Du et al., 2007; Singh et al., 2006). The results obtained with cortical thickness analysis are in agreement with data obtained measuring grey matter volume, and shown a higher sensitivity to subtle changes, therefore ideal for the very early disease phase.

Recently, a variety of other imaging techniques, in addition to the conventional structural techniques, have been evaluated regarding their usefulness as diagnostic or prognostic biomarkers in AD. Some of these new techniques have shown very promising results; further studies allowing for rigorous assessment of test–retest reliability, power calculations, and cost effectiveness, in comparison with the established techniques, are necessary.

In particular, we will briefly summarize data obtained with the Diffusion Tensor Imaging (DTI) technique. DTI is sensitive to the degree of microscopic motion of water molecules. In tissues, this motion is hindered by the physical boundaries of the 3-dimensional tissue microstructure and thus occurs preferentially perpendicular to those boundaries. In highly structured tissues, e.g., white matter, the motion of the water molecules along the axonal direction becomes anisotropic, and allows identifying fibre tracts. Damage to the tissue microstructure results in a loss of anisotropy, which can be detected by DTI.

DTI has been used to identify age-related brain changes (Salat et al., 2005) and white matter alterations in a number of neurodegenerative disorders including AD (Catani, 2006). DTI abnormalities in AD were found in the corpus callosum, and in the white matter of the parietal, temporal, and occipital lobes, posterior cingulate, and hippocampus (Fellgiebel et al., 2004; Head et al., 2004; Kantarci et al., 2005; Taoka et al., 2006).

Although it is most likely that reduced anisotropy within the white matter is secondary to cortical neuronal degeneration, comparative DTI and postmortem pathological studies are necessary to understand the contribution of a primary white matter pathology to these changes (Catani, 2006).

DTI tractography has been used to localize fractional anisotropy changes within specific networks in ageing and AD. In AD, tract-specific measurements show fractional anisotropy changes within long range association tracts of the temporal lobe but no changes in the visual radiations (Taoka et al., 2006). Sullivan and colleagues used tract-specific measurements to show ageing-related reduction of fractional anisotropy within fibres of the corpus callosum (Sullivan et al., 2006). These changes correlated with performances in the Stroop task, and were more evident in the frontal portion of the corpus callosum (genu) compared to the posterior portions (e.g. splenium). Although loss of white matter is prominent in later stages of the neurodegenerative process, preliminary DTI studies in AD found fractional anisotropy reduction in vulnerable white matter regions even at preclinical stages. For example DTI of the corpus callosum and medial temporal lobe revealed that an increased genetic risk for developing AD (ApoE4 carriers) is associated with reduced fractional anisotropy well before the onset of dementia (Persson et al., 2006). In subjects with amnesic MCI, DTI-derived measures from a left hippocampal region-of-interest demonstrate higher sensitivity (around 80%) than volume measurements of hippocampal atrophy (50%) (Müller et al., 2007). These changes are probably related to the underlying pathology as suggested by significant correlations between neuropsychological assessment scores and regional DTI measures in MCI (Rose et al., 2006). An increased water diffusivity in the hippocampus was found to be useful not only for discrimination between AD and healthy controls but also for discrimination between MCI and healthy controls and prediction of cognitive decline in MCI (Kantarci et al., 2001; Kantarci et al., 2005). Patterns of fibre tracts reductions appear also to be specific for the ongoing neurodegenerative process, as shown in recent papers on dementias, such as LBD and FTLD (Borroni et al., 2007; Borroni et al., 2008; Bozzali et al., 2005; Padovani et al., 2006).

3.2. Functional MRI

3.2.1. Functional Magnetic Resonance Imaging (fMRI)

Functional magnetic resonance imaging (fMRI) is a tool that by exploiting the principles of traditional MRI, allows visualizing regional brain activity non-invasively. Although the exact mechanisms underlying the coupling between neural function and fMRI signal changes remain unclear, fMRI studies have been successful in confirming task-specific activation in a variety of brain regions, providing converging evidence for functional localization. In particular, fMRI methods based on blood oxygenation level dependent (BOLD) contrast and arterial spin labelling (ASL) perfusion contrast have enabled imaging of changes in blood oxygenation and cerebral blood flow (CBF).

While BOLD contrast has been widely used as the surrogate marker for neural activation and can provide reliable information on the neuroanatomy underlying transient sensorimotor and cognitive functions, DSW and ASL imaging are mostly used for resting state perfusion measurements (Detre and Wang, 2002).

Bold

In response to neural activation, there is an increased rCBF to the relevant region, but for reasons that are still not well understood, the rCBF increases far more (by 30-50%) than the expected increase in oxygen demand (oxygen extraction increases by only 5%.) (Ogawa et al., 1990). This leads to both local increase of oxyhaemoglobin concentration, which has diamagnetic properties, and reduction of deoxyhaemoglobin, which has paramagnetic properties. The presence of paramagnetic substances in the blood could act as vascular markers, featuring as natural endogenous contrast agent. As such, the BOLD signal is an indirect marker of brain activity, as it evaluates only haemodynamic changes, and usually peaks with a delay of 6-9 seconds (Logothetis and Pfeuffer, 2004; Logothetis and Wandell, 2004; Logothetis et al., 2001).

fMRI has advantages in spatial and temporal resolution when compared to the PET technique, and, in addition, the fact that no radionuclides are used makes it feasible to repeat experiments several times on the same subject. However, fMRI imaging has some limits. The main limit is that MRI does not allow molecular imaging, as compared with Emission Tomography techniques. Also, there are interferences with the magnetic field in some structures of the brain, in particular the orbito-frontal, inferior temporal regions and the temporal pole, because of the air enclosed in adjacent structures (the middle ear and the mastoid bone), resulting in a loss of signal detection (Gorno-Tempini et al., 2002).

Currently, fMRI activation studies are mostly used to gain a better understanding of the neuronal networks involved in specific tasks in the healthy human brain. Much of the recent neuroimaging research on ageing has focused on investigating the relationship between age-related changes in brain structure/function and concomitant changes in cognitive/behavioural abilities. Memory impairment is one of the hallmarks of ageing, and the majority of neuroimaging studies in this area have focused on age-related changes during working memory (WM) and episodic memory (EM) task performance (Craik and Salthouse, 2000). Age-related deficits in WM and EM abilities are related to changes in prefrontal cortex (PFC) function (Cabeza and Nyberg, 2005; Gazzaley et al., 2005; Persson et al., 2006). Noteworthy, these age-related changes in PFC activity were associated either with poorer performance of older subjects or with an absence of behavioural differences between elderly and young subjects (Rypma and D'Esposito, 2000).

Reviews of these neuroimaging studies have generally concluded that with age there is a reduction in the hemispheric specialization of cognitive function in the frontal lobes and viewed the PFC as a homogeneous region. For example, Cabeza (2002) proposed the hemispheric asymmetry reduction in old adults (HAROLD) model, which has been supported by subsequent experimental findings (Cabeza, 2002). However, this model does not address whether these laterality effects are specific to particular brain regions or common to all brain regions and does not specify the underlying neural mechanisms for age-related reductions in lateralized activity. A comprehensive qualitative meta-analytic review of all the fMRI and PET ageing studies of WM and episodic memory that report PFC activation, indicates that in normal ageing distinct PFC regions exhibit different patterns of functional change, suggesting that age-related changes in PFC function are not homogeneous in nature (Rajah and D'Esposito, 2005). Specifically, the effects of ageing that are related to neural degeneration and changes in neurotransmitter systems, will result both in functional deficits and in dedifferentiation of cortical function. These changes in turn result in functional compensation within other PFC regions.

Only a minority of studies addresses the question of how these networks are altered in subjects at risk for AD (MCI) or in subjects with very early AD. Studies conducted in patients with a clinical diagnosis of AD consistently show that medial temporal lobe activation is decreased in comparison to older controls (Machulda et al., 2003; Small et al., 1999).

Some fMRI studies concern subjects whose cognitive function falls between that of normal aging and mild AD, as in MCI, and the results so far have been inconsistent (Dickerson et al., 2004; Machulda et al., 2003; Small et al., 1999). MCI is a heterogeneous condition and this clinical heterogeneity may, in part, explain differences among previous fMRI studies of MCI. An fMRI study investigated whether hippocampal and entorhinal activation during learning is altered in the earliest phase of mild cognitive impairment. The subjects with MCI performed similarly to controls on the fMRI recognition memory task, whereas patients with AD had poorer performance. There were no differences in hippocampal or entorhinal volumes, but significantly greater hippocampal activation was present in the MCI group compared to controls. In contrast, the AD group showed hippocampal and entorhinal hypoactivation and atrophy in comparison to controls. The authors hypothesize that there is a phase of increased medial temporal lobe activation early in the course of prodromal AD followed by a subsequent decrease as the disease progresses (Dickerson et al., 2005).

The results of cognitive activation studies in aging and MCI are complex to interpret, however, an important contribution is already starting to become clear. The largely implicit logic, which tended to associate a larger activation with a better performance, is clearly questionable. The situation appears to be more complex, with evidence of rearrangements and recruitment of additional resources in order to support performance (D'Esposito et al., 2003). Whereas such studies unquestionably give interesting insights into functional deficits and compensatory mechanisms in AD, they might be less suited as diagnostic or prognostic biomarkers because they depend very much on the compliance of the subject.

ASL and DWI

In the last few years, different MR techniques to measure brain perfusion have been developed. ASL and Dynamic susceptibility weighted (DSW) MRI are based on the principle that the passage of contrast material through the tissue microvasculature results in signal intensity changes in T2-weighted images. DSW uses an exogenous paramagnetic contrast, while ASL methods are based on the same principle but use an endogenous tracer, i.e., blood water molecules in arteries providing the blood flow to the brain are "magnetically tagged." These tagged water molecules then diffuse across the blood–brain barrier into the brain and alter the local magnetization state of the brain tissue in proportion to the inflow of saturated protons.

Like emission tomography techniques, both ASL and DWI have shown regions of hypoperfusion in the temporo-parietal lobes and in the posterior cingulate in AD and MCI (Bozzao et al., 2001; Harris et al., 1996; Johnson et al., 2005).

A recent work has investigated ASL MRI for detecting pattern of hypoperfusion in frontotemporal dementia (FTD) and AD vs. cognitively normal control subjects, and found specific hypoperfusion in right frontal regions in patients with FTD vs. control subjects, and a higher perfusion than AD in the parietal regions and posterior cingulate: with further development and evaluation, arterial spin labelling MRI could contribute to the differential diagnosis between frontotemporal dementia and AD (Du et al., 2006).

However, further studies are still required to test the applicability of these methods also for quantification purposes and in studies of single subjects, as compared with the extensively validated emission tomography techniques.

3.2.2. PET and SPECT

The imaging methods of positron emission tomography (PET) and single photon emission computed tomography (SPECT) allow the *in vivo* measurement of several parameters of brain function. These methods are sensitive to modifications taking place at the cellular level, which are not necessarily reflected in morphological abnormalities. They are thus providing a different type of information, in comparison with structural and functional imaging such as provided by MRI.

These include oxygenation levels, perfusion, metabolism, and also neurotransmission. Noteworthy, radiolabelled tracers for receptor occupancy or enzymatic activities represent a unique tool for the *in vivo* measurement of specific neurotransmission systems. Direct measures of therapeutic targets by PET may provide unique information on drug action in vivo, allowing studies of the effects in selected patient populations (Halldin et al., 2001).

Differences between PET and SPECT depend on the properties of positron and gamma emissions. The emission, for each event, of two positrons with a relative angle of 180°, is the physical basis of the PET detection system, and allows greater resolution. The availability of positron emitting radioisotopes, such as carbon, oxygen and fluorine, which can fit into biologically relevant molecules without altering their biological properties, allows the synthesis of PET tracers or radiopharmaceuticals that closely share the properties of normally occurring brain substances. These two factors give PET substantial advantages. On the other hand, the main advantage of the SPECT technique consist in its lower costs and consequent wider availability.

PET can provide steady-state measurements of brain functional parameters, such as oxygen consumption by inhaling $^{15}O_2$, or glucose metabolism and blood flow by i.v. injection of ^{18}F-2-fluoro-2-deoxy-D-glucose (FDG), and radioactive labelled water ($H_2^{15}O$), respectively. $H_2^{15}O$ with PET is also used in functional activation studies to evaluate regional cerebral blood flow changes associated with cognitive performances.

PET radiolabelled tracers allow measuring receptors alterations, in particular dopaminergic and serotoninergic ones, as well as for enzymatic activity and receptors occupancy by drugs (i.e. neuroleptics). For example, dopadecarboxylase enzymatic activity can be measured by ^{18}F-DOPA, acetylcholinesterase activity by ^{11}C-MP4A, post-synaptic dopamine receptor density by ^{11}C-raclopride, and presynaptic dopamine activity by ^{11}C-FECIT.

SPECT results partially parallel those obtained with PET when related biochemical processes (i.e. regional cerebral blood flow, neurotransmission parameters) are examined. SPECT imaging, however, has a lower spatial resolution, a lower signal-to-noise ratio, and ^{123}Iodine or ^{99m}Technetium, the most commonly used isotopes, have a longer half-life and have a structure which is likely to change the ligand's chemical properties.

SPECT is especially used for "cerebral blood-flow" studies, for which two ligands are commercially available, hexamethyl-propylene amine oxime (HMPAO) and N'-1, 2-ethylenediy (bis-L-cysteine) diethyl ester (ECD), and for measuring dopaminergic degeneration in PD and parkinsonisms with the presynaptic dopaminergic ligand FP-CIT (McKeith et al., 2007; Walker et al., 1999).

Brain Perfusion and Brain Metabolism

PET and SPECT are playing an increasing role in the investigation of AD and other degenerative conditions (Herholz et al., 1993; Herholz et al., 2002). The loss of synaptic activity occurring in AD is readily reflected in regional decreases of cerebral metabolic activity and blood flow that are not simply a consequence of tissue loss.

The reduction of metabolism has a characteristic topographic distribution, involving the associative cortex in the temporo-parietal areas of both hemispheres, with the angular gyrus usually being the centre of the metabolic impairment (Herholz et al., 2002; Hoffman et al., 2000). Frontolateral association cortex is also frequently involved to a variable degree (Haxby et al., 1988; Herholz et al., 2002). Primary motor, somatosensory and visual cortical areas are relatively spared. This pattern corresponds in general to the clinical symptoms, with impairment of memory and high-order cognition, including complex perceptual processing and planning of action, but with relative preservation of primary motor and sensory function. These changes differ from those of normal aging, which leads to predominantly medial frontal metabolic decline and may cause some apparent dorsal parietal and frontotemporal (perisylvian) metabolic reduction due to partial volume effects caused by atrophy (Moeller et al., 1996; Petit-Taboué et al., 1998; Zuendorf et al., 2003). The hypometabolism appears to be related to amyloid deposition, at least in areas which are still metabolically viable (Mega et al., 1999). The histochemical correlate of reduced FDG uptake is a pronounced decline in cytochrome oxidase activity in AD relative to controls, whereas adjacent motor cortex does not show such differences (Valla et al., 2001).

Longitudinal studies have shown that the severity and extent of metabolic impairment in temporal and parietal cortex increases as dementia progresses, and frontal involvement becomes more prominent (Mielke et al., 1994). The decline of metabolism is in the order of 16 to 19% over 3 years in association cortices, which contrasts with an absence of significant decline in normal control subjects (Smith et al., 1992). Metabolic rates in basal ganglia and thalamus remain stable and are unrelated to progression (Smith et al., 1992).

In particular, a prospective study of FDG PET has addressed the issue of progression rate of AD, and found that impairment of glucose metabolism in temporo-parietal or frontal association areas measured with PET is significantly associated with dementia severity, clinical classification as possible vs. probable AD, presence of multiple cognitive deficits, and history of progression, and a prognostic indicator of clinical deterioration during follow-up (Herholz et al., 1999). The correlation between initial metabolic ratio and subsequent decline of MMSE score during follow-up is particularly evident in mildly affected patients. Thus, impairment of glucose metabolism in temporo-parietal and frontal association cortex is not only an indicator of dementia severity, but also predicts progression of clinical symptoms (Herholz et al., 1999).

Methods for automatic detection of abnormal metabolism on individual PET scans, providing unbiased measurements, have also been developed. They require appropriate reference data sets, spatial normalization of scans, and statistical algorithms to compare the voxels in scan data with normal reference data, and suitable display of the results. Signorini and colleagues demonstrated that this can be achieved by adapting the Statistical Parametric Mapping (SPM) software package (Signorini et al., 1999). Some commercial software packages provide similar approaches, but users should take care to check the validity of normal reference data, statistics and normalization procedures. Studies that used voxel-based comparisons to normal reference data clearly showed that the posterior cingulate gyrus and the precuneus are also impaired early in AD (Minoshima et al., 1997). Thus, this potential diagnostic sign is easily detected by automated analysis of FDG PET scans. An example of SPM analysis in a single subject with early AD is provided in Figure 2.

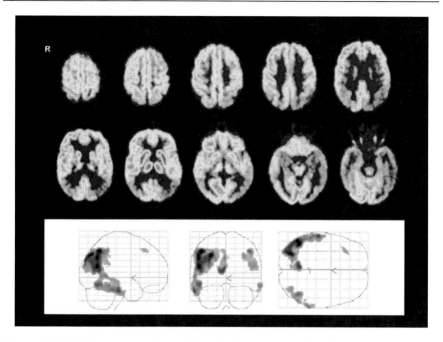

Figure 2. FDG-PET scan in a subject with early AD (upper panel), and Statistical Parametric Mapping comparison of the same PET scan with a group of healthy controls (lower panel). The images show the typical pattern of hypometabolism, involving temporoparietal association cortices, and precuneus. See text for details.

Other approaches has been proposed for the detection of abnormal voxels, aiming at the automatic recognition of the typical metabolic abnormalities in AD. For example, discriminant functions derived by multiple regression of regional data achieved 87% correct classification of AD patients versus controls (Azari et al., 1993), and a neural network classifier arrived at 90% accuracy (Kippenhan et al., 1994). The sum of abnormal t-values in regions that are typically hypometabolic in AD has been used as an indicator with 93% accuracy (Herholz et al., 2002). Patients with late-onset AD may show less difference between typically affected and non-affected brain regions than usually seen in early-onset AD, which could potentially lead to reduced diagnostic accuracy with FDG PET (Mosconi, 2005).

The main contribution of these methods is the ability to identify changes that occur in single subjects and to describe pattern that orient and confirm clinical diagnosis.

According to neuropathological studies, the earliest pathological changes in AD develop in the transentorhinal and entorhinal regions, then spread to the hippocampus and finally towards the neocortex. Medial temporal reduction in metabolism can thus be expected to be the earliest markers of the disease process. Yamaguchi and colleagues (1997) have shown that the reduction in cortical metabolism is significantly correlated with hippocampal atrophy, as shown with structural MR (Yamaguchi et al., 1997). Atrophy of hippocampus and parahippocampal structures is a main finding of structural imaging in AD. Therefore, one would expect also major functional changes of glucose metabolism in this brain area, but this has not generally been the case (Ishii et al., 1998). It is difficult to identify hippocampal metabolic impairment on FDG PET scans, because this region has lower resting metabolism than neocortex, and pathological changes are not obvious by visual image analysis. However, by coregistration with MRI for accurate positioning of regions of interest onto the hippocampus in FDG PET scans a reduction especially of entorhinal metabolism has indeed been observed in MCI and AD (Mosconi et al., 2005). In addition, in normal controls, glucose metabolism in neocortex is correlated with entorhinal cortex across both hemispheres, whereas in AD patients these correlations are largely lost (Mosconi et al., 2004).

The observation that medial temporal lobe damage leads also to mnemonic dysfunction have been advanced greatly by the study of neurodegenerative disorders' patients. In AD, the study of the correlations between memory test scores and metabolic values across a sample of subjects provided a map of those brain structures whose synaptic dysfunction underlies the particular neuropsychological alteration. The distribution of the sites of correlations with specific memory deficits shows striking differences according to which memory system is involved and to the severity of the impairment (Desgranges et al., 2002; Eustache et al., 2000). In fact, significant correlations involved bilaterally not only several limbic structures (the hippocampal/entorhinal cortex regions, posterior cingulate gyrus and retrosplenial cortex), but also some temporo-occipital association areas. In the less severe subgroup, all significant correlations were restricted to the parahippocampal gyrus and retrosplenial cortex, in accordance with the known involvement of this network in normal and impaired memory function, while in the more severe subgroup they mainly involved the left temporal neocortex, which is known to be implicated in semantic memory. The authors suggest that, when episodic memory is mildly impaired, limbic functions are still sufficient to subserve the remaining performance, whereas with more severe memory deficit resulting from accumulated pathology, the neocortical areas become more functionally involved (Desgranges et al., 2002). This approach opens the way for the unravelling of the neurobiological substrates of both cognitive impairment and compensatory mechanisms in neurological diseases. Such studies in brain-diseased subjects are particularly useful for establishing cognitive and neurobiological models of human memory, because they allow the highlighting of the neural networks that are essential for memory function.

Furthermore, imaging with FDG and PET might also allow identifying the so-called brain reserve. The concept of cognitive or cerebral reserve ("brain reserve hypothesis") is based on the clinical observation that highly intelligent or educated individuals appear to be able to cope better with the onset of dementia, maintaining a normal functional level for a longer time than less educated people (Christensen et al., 2007; Stern et al., 1992; Stern, 2002). This observation is documented by neuropathological and epidemiological studies (Bennett et al., 2003; Goldman et al., 2001; Ince, 2001; McDowell et al., 2007; Ngandu et al., 2007; Roe et al., 2007; Scarmeas et al., 2006; Snowdon et al., 1989)

FDG PET data provide supporting evidences, demonstrating that there is a significant inverse relationship between educational/occupational level and regional glucose metabolism in the posterior temporo-parietal association cortex and the precuneus in AD (see Figure 3), showing that the level of education and occupation provides a functional reserve capacity probably contrasting the clinical onset and progression of dementia (Garibotto et al., in press; Perneczky et al., 2006).

Even at an asymptomatic stage, impairment of cortical glucose metabolism has been observed in preclinical stage in subjects at high risk for AD due to family history of AD and ApoE4 homozygosis (Reiman et al., 2004; Small et al., 2000). In middle-aged and elderly asymptomatic ApoE4-positive subjects temporoparietal and posterior cingulate glucose metabolism declines by about 2% per year (Reiman et al., 1996).

Data are accumulating that the presence of the AD metabolic pattern in MCI predicts conversion to clinical dementia of Alzheimer type, and therefore indicates "incipient AD". Non-demented patients with mild cognitive impairment may indeed show metabolic impairment of association cortices, which is characteristic of AD. MCI patient groups when compared to normal controls typically show significantly impaired metabolism (Minoshima et al., 1997). Anchisi and colleagues have demonstrated that by neuropsychological testing alone one can identify subjects who are likely not to progress to dementia because their memory deficit is relatively mild, thus providing a high negative predictive value with regard to progression. However, prediction based on neuropsychological testing is less reliable for MCI patients with more severe memory impairment.

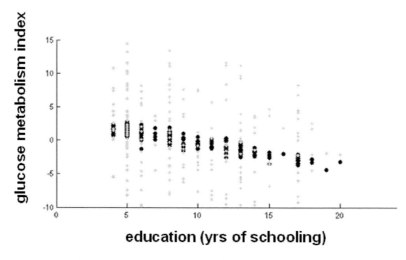

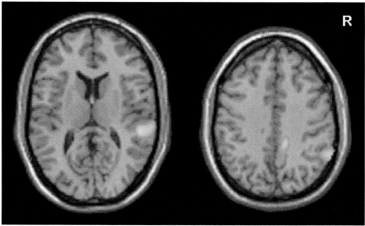

Figure 3. Brain reserve provided by education in a group of subjects with early AD. Upper panel shows the significant inverse correlation of education and brain glucose metabolism, located in the precuneus and left temporoparietal cortex, as shown in the lower panel. See text for details.

In these patients FDG PET adds significant information by separating those who will progress within the next twelve months from those who will remain stable (Anchisi et al., 2005). Similar evidences have been obtained measuring brain perfusion with SPECT, and comparing patterns of hypoperfusion across groups (Borroni et al., 2006). The relative hypometabolism observed in MCI converters, as compared with MCI non-converters, is shown in Figure 4.

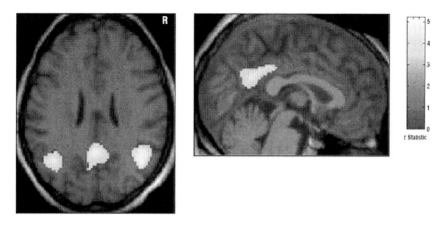

Figure 4. Hypometabolism in posterior cingulate cortex/precuneus, in a group of MCI converters, as compared with healthy age matched controls. See text for details.

Depending on subject selection, functional neuroimaging has thus a prognostic impact. A longitudinal study of cognitively normal subjects indicated that cognitive decline to MCI within 3-years follow-up is related to metabolic reductions in entorhinal cortex at entry, independent of ε4 status (Mosconi et al., 2005).

Few studies so far compared FDG PET with other biomarkers. In a study, PET prediction accuracy was best (94%) within the ApoE4 group (Mosconi et al., 2004). In another report, MCI subjects were followed over 16 months, the positive and negative predictive values of FDG PET for progression to AD were 85% and 94%, respectively, whereas corresponding values for the ApoE4 genotype were 53% and 77% only (Drzezga et al., 2005). By combination of the two indicators, predictive values increased to 100% in subgroups of patients with concurrent genetic and metabolic findings. When comparing phosphorylated tau protein in CSF with FDG PET in MCI, Fellgiebl and colleagues found similar findings with both tests (Fellgiebel et al., 2004). Some studies indicate that combining targeted neuropsychology testing, platelet amyloid precursor protein ratio with SPECT (Borroni et al., 2005) may reach a prediction accuracy even close to 90%.

Not only PET and SPECT represent a supportive tool for early dementia diagnosis, but also in differential diagnosis between AD and FTD. Many studies have indeed used these techniques to compare AD with other forms of dementia. Recent evidences support the validity of emission tomography techniques to differentiate AD patients and FTLD patients, and its superiority to clinical diagnosis alone (Foster et al., 2007; McNeill et al., 2007).

PET and SPECT might be very useful in supporting differential diagnosis in LBD, which is recognized as the second most common form of neurodegenerative dementia, and has been found to have substantial pathologic and clinical overlap with AD (Hansen et al., 1993; McKeith et al., 1996).

Neuroimaging findings indicate a relative preservation of glucose metabolism and rCBF in medial temporal lobe structures in LBD (Colloby et al., 2002). Several studies also indicate differences in perfusion patterns on SPECT or fluorodeoxyglucose PET with a selective occipital hypoperfusion or hypometabolism in LBD compared with AD (Ishii et al., 2007; Minoshima et al., 2001; Pasquier et al., 2002). Minoshima and colleagues presented high discrimination accuracy of 90% sensitivity and 80% specificity between AD and LBD considering hypometabolism in the occipital cortex (Minoshima et al., 2001). Reduced occipital activity has been recognized as a supportive feature in the diagnosis of LBD (McKeith et al., 2005).

Finally, the diagnosis of Vascular Dementia (VD) is normally made by a combination of history, neurologic examination, and MRI. SPECT and PET are usually only needed for equivocal cases. However, 15%–20% of demented patients will have a mixed dementia, most often VD and AD (Gold et al., 2007). In such cases, SPECT or PET imaging is useful to distinguish between AD alone, VD alone, and a mixed dementia. Talbot and colleagues studied 363 patients with dementia (AD =132, VD =78, LBD =24, FTD =58, progressive aphasia =22) and calculated likelihood ratios for various pairwise disease group comparisons in order to determine the degree to which different patterns of rCBF found on initial SPECT imaging modify clinical diagnoses. Bilateral posterior temporoparietal defects significantly increased the odds of a patient having AD as opposed to VD or FTD. Bilateral anterior abnormalities significantly increased the odds of having FTD as opposed to AD or LBD. "Patchy" defects significantly increased the odds of having VD relative to AD. (Talbot et al., 1998). Likelihood ratios reported by Talbot and colleagues are similar to those reported by Jagust and colleagues (Jagust et al., 2001). Kerrouche and colleagues recently validated a voxel-based multivariate technique to a large FDG PET data set, and showed that lower metabolism differentiating VD from AD mainly concerned the deep grey nuclei, cerebellum, primary cortices, middle temporal gyrus, and anterior cingulate gyrus, whereas lower metabolism in AD versus VD concerned mainly the hippocampal region and orbitofrontal, posterior cingulate, and posterior parietal cortices. (Kerrouche et al., 2006).

The impact of functional neuroimaging in the diagnostic and prognostic management of AD has been recognized also in many recently published guidelines of neurological societies (Dubois et al., 2007; Knopman et al., 2001; Waldemar et al., 2007).

The paper by Knopman and colleagues reported an evidence-based review of the parameters for diagnosis of dementia: they state that both PET and SPECT imaging provided promising results, for diagnosis confirmation as well as differential diagnosis (Knopman et al., 2001).

The last European Federation of Neurological Societies guidelines recommends the usage of SPECT and PET in those cases where diagnostic uncertainty remains after clinical and structural imaging work up (Waldemar et al., 2007).

Most importantly, the revised NINCDS-ADRDA criteria definitely confirm and state the usefulness of biomarkers, including also neuroimaging: the diagnostic criteria are centred on a clinical core of early and significant episodic memory impairment, but there must also be at least one or more abnormal biomarkers among structural neuroimaging with MRI, molecular neuroimaging with PET, and cerebrospinal fluid analysis of amyloid β or tau proteins (Dubois et al., 2007).

Brain Amyloid Deposition

A recent and very interesting progress for neuroimaging in AD is represented by the development of new tracers that bind with high affinity to fibrillar amyloid plaques and thus allow for the first time an in vivo quantification of the amyloid burden (Cai et al., 2007; Nordberg, 2004).

The first tested in humans is the [11]C Pittsburgh Compound-B (^{11}C-PIB) , binding selectively to amyloid plaques (Klunk et al., 2004). A recent report showed in AD a typical retention in areas of association cortex known to contain large amounts of amyloid deposits in AD, most prominently in frontal cortex (1.94-fold, p = 0.0001), and also in parietal (1.71-fold, p = 0.0002), temporal (1.52-fold, p = 0.002), and occipital (1.54-fold, p = 0.002) cortex and the striatum (1.76-fold, p = 0.0001). ^{11}C-PIB retention was equivalent in AD patients and controls in areas known to be relatively unaffected by amyloid deposition (such as subcortical white matter, pons, and cerebellum). In cortical areas, ^{11}C-PIB retention correlated inversely with cerebral glucose metabolism determined with FDG (Klunk et al., 2004).

The second attempt in patients with AD to detect in vivo abnormal amyloid deposition in the brain used instead is a radiofluorinated compound (^{18}F-FDDNP) that binds to amyloid plaques but also to neurofibrillary tangles and to prion plaques in human autopsy brain tissue (Agdeppa et al., 2001; Agdeppa et al., 2003; Bresjanac et al., 2003).

The studies by Shoghi-Jadid and co-workers found retention in the temporal, parietal, frontal, and occipital cortical regions of the AD patients, 10–15% higher than in the pons. The highest retention of ^{18}F-FDDNP in the patients was observed in the hippocampus, amygdala, and entorhinal cortex where the retention was 30% higher than in the pons (Shoghi-Jadid et al., 2002). A negative correlation was observed between binding of ^{18}F-FDDNP and cognitive status of the patients with AD (Kepe et al., 2006).

This new tracer class has not only the potential to improve the accuracy of the diagnosis of AD, but also allows to study the effects of various kinds of treatments on one of the histological hallmarks of the disease. Early detection of pathological changes such as amyloid deposition in AD will be a prerequisite for early treatment, and in vivo imaging represents the ideal instrument to assess the effectiveness of antiamyloid therapy.

A recent study assessed beta amyloid deposition in MCI, and found values intermediate between those obtained in healthy controls and in AD patients, and significantly different from both groups (Small et al., 2006). Therefore, amyloid imaging can differentiate persons with MCI from those with AD and those with no cognitive impairment.

A prospective study in MCI has demonstrated that those MCI subjects that later at clinical follow-up converted to AD showed significant higher PIB retention compared to non-converting MCI patients and HC, with a PIB retention comparable to AD patients (Forsberg et al., in press). Correlations were observed in the MCI patients between PIB retention and CSF Aß1-42, total Tau and episodic memory scores, respectively (Forsberg et al., in press).

An interesting perspective is suggested by a recent work (Pike et al., 2007). Beta amyloid deposition may occur also in normal elderly people without apparent cognitive effect. The authors examined this relationship using ^{11}C-PIB PET vivo in healthy ageing (HA), MCI and AD. Ninety-seven percent of AD, 61% of MCI and 22% of HA cases had increased cortical ^{11}C-PIB binding, indicating the presence of Abeta plaques. There was a strong relationship between impaired episodic memory performance and ^{11}C-PIB binding, both in MCI and HA. This relationship was weaker in AD and less robust for non-memory cognitive domains. Therefore, Abeta deposition in the asymptomatic elderly is associated with episodic memory impairment. This finding, together with the strong relationship between ^{11}C-PIB binding and the severity of memory impairment in MCI, suggests that individuals with increased cortical ^{11}C-PIB binding are on the path to AD. Early intervention trials for AD targeted to non-demented individuals with cerebral Abeta deposition are warranted.

Amyloid imaging has been recently tested also for its potential in the differential diagnosis of dementia. Preliminary data show that Semantic Dementia (Drzezga et al., 2008) and Parkinson's Disease Dementia (Maetzler et al., 2007) have a significantly lower PIB retention, as compared with AD.

Neurochemical Imaging in AD

Neurochemical imaging is one of the most established "molecular" imaging techniques. There have been tremendous efforts expended to develop radioligands specific to various neurochemical system. Investigational applications of neurochemical imaging in dementing disorders are extensive. Cholinergic, dopaminergic, and serotoninergic systems, as well as benzodiazepine receptors, opioid receptors, and glutamatergic receptors have been imaged in AD and other dementing disorders. These investigations have provided important insights into disease processes in living human patients (see for a review Minoshima et al., 2004).

We will focus mainly on the first two systems, cholinergic and dopaminergic, which have the stronger impact in the clinical management and differential diagnosis of dementias.

Brain Acetylcholinesterase Activity

The first group encompasses carbon 11–labelled acetylcholine analogues, which allow for an in vivo measurement of the activity of the acetylcholine degrading enzyme acetylcholinesterase (ACHE), such as ^{11}C-MP4A. AD is associated with loss of cholinergic neurons in the basal fore-brain and, thus, with decreased levels of acetylcholine and the enzymes responsible for its synthesis and degradation in this region and connected cortical regions. In accordance with this, several PET studies have found a reduction of the cortical ACHE activity in AD compared with controls, particularly in the hippocampus and parieto-temporal regions (Herholz et al., 2004; Iyo et al., 1997; Shinotoh et al., 2000).

The degree of the ACHE reduction was found to be well correlated with the degree of the cognitive impairment (Bohnen et al., 2005). Furthermore, treatment with ACHE inhibitors resulted in a measurable decrease of the remaining ACHE activity and was well correlated with improvements of the cognitive measures (Kuhl et al., 2000; Shinotoh et al., 2001). Therefore, this technique seems to be quite promising not only as a diagnostic biomarker but also as a prognostic biomarker.

However, a validation of these data in larger cohort of subjects is required, to test the diagnostic and prognostic potential of ACHE evaluation, and for this goal multicentre european studies included in the DIMI network are ongoing (see the Research in progress section).

With ^{11}C-MP4A imaging of acetylcholinesterase activity and PET, Rinne and colleagues found only a slight hippocampal acetylcholinesterase activity reduction in MCI and early AD subjects, concluding that the value of in vivo acetylcholinesterase measurements in detecting the early AD process is limited (Rinne et al., 2003).

On the contrary, Herholz and colleagues found a significant reduction of ^{11}C-MP4A in 3 MCI, out of a 8 subjects' group, and a significant association was found with progression to AD within 18 months, suggesting that low cortical acetylcholinesterase activity may be an indicator of impending dementia in patients with mild cognitive impairment (Herholz et al., 2005).

Brain Dopaminergic Transmission

Neurochemical correlates of extrapyramidal symptoms frequently observed in AD are not understood fully. A postmortem investigation suggested a correlation between neurofibrillary tangle density in the substantia nigra and extrapyramidal signs in AD (Liu et al., 1997). Dopaminergic imaging of dementing disorders can thus increase our understanding of the neuronal correlates of cognitive as well as motor impairments in various dementing disorders.

This issue became a focus of PET and SPECT investigations. A study using ^{18}F-fluorodopa PET indicated no significant reduction in ^{18}F-fluorodopa uptake in the caudate or putamen of rigid or non-rigid patients with AD versus normal controls. In contrast, there were severe reductions in PD, indicating differential underlying mechanisms of extrapyramidal symptoms in AD and PD (Tyrrell et al., 1990). The ^{123}I-IBZM SPECT showed modest striatal D_2 receptor reductions of approximately 15% in AD without overt extrapyramidal signs, in comparison to controls. This result suggested a decline of postsynaptic striatal dopamine receptors as a part of AD pathophysiology that is different from prevalent presynaptic nigrostriatal degeneration (Pizzolato et al., 1996). In contrast, subsequent dopamine transporter imaging using a cocaine analogue, 2-ß-carbomethoxy-3-ß-(4-^{18}F-fluorophenyl) tropane (ß-CFT), showed more severe reductions in the putamen or caudate in patients with AD with extrapyramidal symptoms (Rinne et al., 1998).

A further PET investigation using a dopamine D_1 receptor antagonist, ^{11}C-NNC 756, and a D_2 antagonist, ^{11}C-raclopride, showed 14% reductions in D_1 receptors in AD but no significant reduction in D_2 receptors (Kemppainen et al., 2000). However, D_1 or D_2 receptor changes did not correlate with Mini Mental State Examination scores or motor Unified PD Rating Scale scores. These imaging investigations indicate differential alterations of dopaminergic markers in AD and PD, but the exact neurochemical basis for extrapyramidal signs in AD requires further investigation.

Dopamine imaging in dementia received much attention in the investigation of LBD. In vivo neurochemical imaging depicted dopaminergic abnormalities in living patients with LBD. Decreased striatal dopamine transporters in LBD was detected using ^{123}I-2-ß-carboxymethoxy-3-ß-[4-iodophenyl]tropane ([123]I-ß-CIT) SPECT (Donnemiller et al., 1997). The caudate/putamen ratio of postsynaptic dopamine D_2 neuroreceptor density measured by IBZM SPECT was significantly lower in probable LBD as compared with probable AD and normal controls (Walker et al., 1997). Decreased binding of dopaminergic presynaptic marker ^{123}I-2-ß-carbomethoxy-3-ß-(4-iodophenyl)-N-(3-fluoropropyl)-nortropane (^{123}I-FP-CIT) was also shown by SPECT in a case of autopsy proven LBD (Walker et al., 1999).

PET using ^{18}F-fluorodopa also showed decreased uptake in the putamen in LBD that distinguished LBD from AD, with a sensitivity of 86% and specificity of 100% (Hu et al., 2000). Decreased ^{18}F-fluorodopa uptake in the putamen measured by PET was also confirmed in an autopsy proven case of pure LBD (Hisanaga et al., 2001). When compared with PD, a more symmetric and severe loss of dopamine transporters was found in LBD (Ransmayr et al., 2001).

Imaging of presynaptic dopaminergic transporters (DAT), with FP-CIT SPECT and ^{11}C-FECIT PET, show significantly low dopamine transporter density in PD and LBD, both in the caudate and putamen, indicating a possible differential diagnosis of LBD from AD (Walker et al., 2002). An example of the ability of DAT imaging to differentiate single cases of AD and LBD is provided in Figure 5.

In particular, a recent multicentre study has investigated the sensitivity and specificity, in the ante-mortem differentiation of probable LBD from other causes of dementia, of single photon emission computed tomography (SPECT) brain imaging with the ligand ^{123}I-FP-CIT (McKeith et al., 2007).

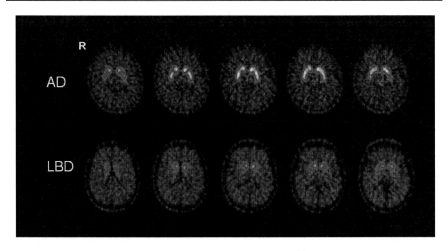

Figure 5. Presynaptic dopamine transporters, as measured by ^{11}C-FECIT and PET, in one subject with AD (upper panel) and one subject with LBD (lower panel). PET images clearly show a pattern of widespread reduction in the LBD patient. See text for details.

Abnormal scans had a mean sensitivity of 77,7% for detecting clinical probable LBD, with specificity of 90,4% for excluding non-LBD dementia, which was predominantly due to AD.

A mean value of 85,7% was achieved for overall diagnostic accuracy, 82,4% for positive predictive value, and 87,5% for negative predictive value. Inter-reader agreement for rating scans as normal or abnormal was high (Cohen's κ=0·87). Therefore, there is a high correlation between abnormal (low binding) DAT activity measured with ^{123}I-FP-CIT SPECT and a clinical diagnosis of probable LBD. The diagnostic accuracy is sufficiently high for this technique to be clinically useful in distinguishing LBD from AD. Low dopamine transporter uptake in basal ganglia demonstrated by PET and SPECT imaging has been suggested as a supportive feature for LBD diagnosis (McKeith et al., 2005).

4. Research in Progress

Over the last years, a number of genetic, biochemical, and imaging measures have been explored regarding potential to improve the accuracy of the clinical diagnosis of AD or to monitor disease progression and treatment effects. Considering the complexity of the AD disease process, it seems also rather unlikely that such a single ideal diagnostic or prognostic AD biomarker even exists. However, as these markers assess slightly different aspects of the disease process, a combination of two or three of them might be much more powerful than each of them alone (Herholz, 2003). Therefore, one of the currently most important issues of clinical AD research is to identify the combination of the already-established biomarkers with the highest diagnostic and prognostic power.

To address these questions, multicentre research projects are ongoing, both in Europe and in the US.

In particular, two active networks are exploring neuroimaging biomarkers of AD and other neurodegenerative disorders:

1. the *Diagnostic and Molecular Imaging Network* (DIMI), launched in June 2005, and connecting many european centres (www.dimi.eu). The DIMI network is funded only by the EU, and the workpackages included aim mainly at addressing translational research from basic science to clinical trials in the identification of novel markers of neurodegeneration and neuroinflammation.

2. the *Alzheimer's Disease Neuroimaging Initiative* (ADNI), launched in October 2004, and connecting many centres in United States and Canada. The ADNI is funded by the National Institute on Aging (NIA) and the National Institute of Biomedical Imaging and Bioengineering (NIBIB) of the National Institutes of Health (NIH), and also by several pharmaceutical companies and foundations (Mueller et al., 2005)

5. Final Remarks

The impact of neuroimaging in the diagnostic and prognostic management of AD has been recognized also in many recently published guidelines of neurological societies (Dubois et al., 2007; Knopman et al., 2001; Waldemar et al., 2007).

The paper by Knopman and colleagues reported an evidence-based review of the parameters for diagnosis of dementia: they concluded that structural neuroimaging with either a noncontrast CT or MR scan in the initial evaluation of patients with dementia is appropriate, at the time of the initial dementia assessment to identify pathology such as brain neoplasms or subdural haematomas, and normal pressure hydrocephalus. Because of insufficient data on validity, no other imaging procedure is recommended, although both PET and SPECT imaging provided promising results, for diagnosis confirmation as well as differential diagnosis (Knopman et al., 2001).

The last European Federation of Neurological Societies guidelines recommends the usage of structural imaging in the evaluation of every patient suspected of dementia: non-contrast CT could help identifying surgically treatable lesions and vascular disease, and, to increase specificity, MRI (with a protocol including T1, T2 and FLAIR sequences) should be used. SPECT and PET may be useful in those cases where diagnostic uncertainty remains after clinical and structural imaging work up, and should not be used as the only imaging measure (Waldemar et al., 2007).

Most importantly, the revised NINCDS-ADRDA criteria definitely confirm and state the usefulness of biomarkers, including also neuroimaging: the diagnostic criteria are centred on a clinical core of early and significant episodic memory impairment, but there must also be at least one or more abnormal biomarkers among structural neuroimaging with MRI, molecular neuroimaging with PET, and cerebrospinal fluid analysis of amyloid β or tau proteins (Dubois et al., 2007).

The timeliness of these criteria is highlighted by the many drugs in development that are directed at changing pathogenesis, particularly at the production and clearance of amyloid β as well as at the hyperphosphorylation state of tau. Validation studies in existing and prospective cohorts are needed to advance these criteria and optimise their sensitivity, specificity, and accuracy (Dubois et al., 2007).

This is an important phase of research in AD in which large longitudinal clinical trials assessing disease modifying interventions are underway.

When disease-modifying treatments become available, biomarkers may prove to be the most effective means of early or predictive diagnosis in the incipient stages of disease and also a mechanism to monitor treatment effects. Neuroimaging, in particular functional and molecular neuroimaging, is surely going to play a central role.

References

Agdeppa, E.D., Kepe, V., Liu, J., Flores-Torres, S., Satyamurthy, N., Petric, A., Cole, G.M., Small, G.W., Huang, S.C., Barrio, J.R., 2001. Binding characteristics of radiofluorinated 6-dialkylamino-2-naphthylethylidene derivatives as positron emission tomography imaging probes for beta-amyloid plaques in Alzheimer's disease. *J Neurosci 21*, RC189.

Agdeppa, E.D., Kepe, V., Liu, J., Small, G.W., Huang, S., Petric, A., Satyamurthy, N., Barrio, J.R., 2003. 2-dialkylamino-6-acylmalononitrile substituted naphthalenes (DDNP analogs): novel diagnostic and therapeutic tools in Alzheimer's disease. *Mol Imaging Biol 5*, 404-417.

Alexander, G.E., Chen, K., Pietrini, P., Rapoport, S.I., Reiman, E.M., 2002. Longitudinal PET evaluation of cerebral metabolic decline in dementia: a potential outcome measure in Alzheimer's disease treatment studies. *Am J Psychiatry 159*, 738-745.

Anchisi, D., Borroni, B., Franceschi, M., Kerrouche, N., Kalbe, E., Beuthien-Beumann, B., Cappa, S., Lenz, O., Ludecke, S., Marcone, A., Mielke, R., Ortelli, P., Padovani, A., Pelati, O., Pupi, A., Scarpini, E., Weisenbach, S., Herholz, K., Salmon, E., Holthoff, V., Sorbi, S., Fazio, F., Perani, D., 2005. Heterogeneity of brain glucose metabolism in mild cognitive impairment and clinical progression to Alzheimer disease. *Arch Neurol 62*, 1728-1733.

Azari, N.P., Pettigrew, K.D., Schapiro, M.B., Haxby, J.V., Grady, C.L., Pietrini, P., Salerno, J.A., Heston, L.L., Rapoport, S.I., Horwitz, B., 1993. Early detection of Alzheimer's disease: a statistical approach using positron emission tomographic data. *J Cereb Blood Flow Metab 13*, 438-447.

Ballmaier, M., O'Brien, J.T., Burton, E.J., Thompson, P.M., Rex, D.E., Narr, K.L., McKeith, I.G., DeLuca, H., Toga, A.W., 2004. Comparing gray matter loss profiles between dementia with Lewy bodies and Alzheimer's disease using cortical pattern matching: diagnosis and gender effects. *Neuroimage 23*, 325-335.

Bennett, D.A., Schneider, J.A., Bienias, J.L., Evans, D.A., Wilson, R.S., 2005. Mild cognitive impairment is related to Alzheimer disease pathology and cerebral infarctions. *Neurology 64*, 834-841.

Bennett, D.A., Wilson, R.S., Schneider, J.A., Evans, D.A., Mendes de Leon, C.F., Arnold, S.E., Barnes, L.L., Bienias, J.L., 2003. Education modifies the relation of AD pathology to level of cognitive function in older persons. *Neurology 60*, 1909-1915.

Bertram, L., Tanzi, R.E., 2004. The current status of Alzheimer's disease genetics: what do we tell the patients? *Pharmacol Res 50*, 385-396.

Bohnen, N.I., Kaufer, D.I., Hendrickson, R., Ivanco, L.S., Lopresti, B., Davis, J.G., Constantine, G., Mathis, C.A., Moore, R.Y., DeKosky, S.T., 2005.

Cognitive correlates of alterations in acetylcholinesterase in Alzheimer's disease. *Neurosci Lett 380*, 127-132.

Borroni, B. and Garibotto, V., Agosti, C., Brambati, S., Zanetti, M., Bellelli, G., Gasparotti, R., Padovani, A., Perani, D., 2008. Structural MRI changes and correlates of limb-apraxia in corticobasal degeneration syndrome: a voxel-based morphometry and diffusion tensor imaging study. *Arch Neurol 65*, 796-801.

Borroni, B., Anchisi, D., Paghera, B., Vicini, B., Kerrouche, N., Garibotto, V., Terzi, A., Vignolo, L.A., Di Luca, M., Giubbini, R., Padovani, A., Perani, D., 2006. Combined 99mTc-ECD SPECT and neuropsychological studies in MCI for the assessment of conversion to AD. *Neurobiol Aging 27*, 24-31.

Borroni, B., Brambati, S.M., Agosti, C., Gipponi, S., Bellelli, G., Gasparotti, R., Garibotto, V., Di Luca, M., Scifo, P., Perani, D., Padovani, A., 2007. Evidence of white matter changes on diffusion tensor imaging in frontotemporal dementia. *Arch Neurol 64*, 246-251.

Borroni, B., Perani, D., Broli, M., Colciaghi, F., Garibotto, V., Paghera, B., Agosti, C., Giubbini, R., Di Luca, M., Padovani, A., 2005. Pre-clinical diagnosis of Alzheimer disease combining platelet amyloid precursor protein ratio and rCBF SPECT analysis. *J Neurol 252*, 1359-1362.

Boxer, A.L., Geschwind, M.D., Belfor, N., Gorno-Tempini, M.L., Schauer, G.F., Miller, B.L., Weiner, M.W., Rosen, H.J., 2006. Patterns of brain atrophy that differentiate corticobasal degeneration syndrome from progressive supranuclear palsy. *Arch Neurol 63*, 81-86.

Bozzali, M., Falini, A., Cercignani, M., Baglio, F., Farina, E., Alberoni, M., Vezzulli, P., Olivotto, F., Mantovani, F., Shallice, T., Scotti, G., Canal, N., Nemni, R., 2005. Brain tissue damage in dementia with Lewy bodies: an in vivo diffusion tensor MRI study. *Brain 128*, 1595-1604.

Bozzao, A., Floris, R., Baviera, M.E., Apruzzese, A., Simonetti, G., 2001. Diffusion and perfusion MR imaging in cases of Alzheimer's disease: correlations with cortical atrophy and lesion load. *AJNR Am J Neuroradiol 22*, 1030-1036.

Braak, H., Braak, E., 1991. Demonstration of amyloid deposits and neurofibrillary changes in whole brain sections. *Brain Pathol 1*, 213-216.

Brambati, S.M., Rankin, K.P., Narvid, J., Seeley, W.W., Dean, D., Rosen, H.J., Miller, B.L., Ashburner, J., Gorno-Tempini, M.L., in press. Atrophy progression in semantic dementia with asymmetric temporal involvement: a tensor-based morphometry study. *Neurobiol Aging* .

Brambati, S.M., Renda, N.C., Rankin, K.P., Rosen, H.J., Seeley, W.W., Ashburner, J., Weiner, M.W., Miller, B.L., Gorno-Tempini, M.L., 2007. A tensor based morphometry study of longitudinal gray matter contraction in FTD. *Neuroimage 35*, 998-1003.

Bresjanac, M., Smid, L.M., Vovko, T.D., Petric, A., Barrio, J.R., Popovic, M., 2003. Molecular-imaging probe 2-(1-[6-[(2-fluoroethyl)(methyl)amino]-2-naphthyl]ethylidene) malononitrile labels prion plaques in vitro. *J Neurosci 23*, 8029-8033.

Burton, E.J., McKeith, I.G., Burn, D.J., Williams, E.D., O'Brien, J.T., 2004. Cerebral atrophy in Parkinson's disease with and without dementia: a comparison with Alzheimer's disease, dementia with Lewy bodies and controls. *Brain 127*, 791-800.

Cabeza, R., 2002. Hemispheric asymmetry reduction in older adults: the HAROLD model. *Psychol Aging 17*, 85-100.

Cabeza, R., Nyberg, L., 2005. Cognitive neuroscience of aging., Oxford University Press.

Cai, L., Innis, R.B., Pike, V.W., 2007. Radioligand development for PET imaging of beta-amyloid (Abeta)--current status. *Curr Med Chem 14*, 19-52.

Catani, M., 2006. Diffusion tensor magnetic resonance imaging tractography in cognitive disorders. *Curr Opin Neurol 19*, 599-606.

Chetelat, G., Baron, J., 2003. Early diagnosis of Alzheimer's disease: contribution of structural neuroimaging. *Neuroimage 18*, 525-541.

Christensen, H., Anstey, K.J., Parslow, R.A., Maller, J., Mackinnon, A., Sachdev, P., 2007. The brain reserve hypothesis, brain atrophy and aging. *Gerontology 53*, 82-95.

Chételat, G., Landeau, B., Eustache, F., Mézenge, F., Viader, F., de la Sayette, V., Desgranges, B., Baron, J., 2005. Using voxel-based morphometry to map the structural changes associated with rapid conversion in MCI: a longitudinal MRI study. *Neuroimage 27*, 934-946.

Colloby, S.J., Fenwick, J.D., Williams, E.D., Paling, S.M., Lobotesis, K., Ballard, C., McKeith, I., O'Brien, J.T., 2002. A comparison of (99m)Tc-HMPAO SPET changes in dementia with Lewy bodies and Alzheimer's disease using statistical parametric mapping. *Eur J Nucl Med Mol Imaging 29*, 615-622.

Craik, F., Salthouse, T., 2000. The handbook of aging and cognition, 2nd ed., Lawrence Erlbaum Associates.

Cummings, J.L., Doody, R., Clark, C., 2007. Disease-modifying therapies for Alzheimer disease: challenges to early intervention. *Neurology 69*, 1622-1634.

D'Esposito, M., Deouell, L., Gazzaley, A., 2003. Alterations in the bold fMRI signal with ageing and disease: a challenge for neuroimaging. *Nat Rev Neurosci 4*, 863-872.

DeKosky, S.T., 2003. Pathology and pathways of Alzheimer's disease with an update on new developments in treatment. *J Am Geriatr Soc 51*, S314-20.

DeKosky, S.T., Marek, K., 2003. Looking backward to move forward: early detection of neurodegenerative disorders. *Science 302*, 830-834.

Desgranges, B., Baron, J., Lalevée, C., Giffard, B., Viader, F., de La Sayette, V., Eustache, F., 2002. The neural substrates of episodic memory impairment in Alzheimer's disease as revealed by FDG-PET: relationship to degree of deterioration. *Brain 125*, 1116-1124.

Detre, J.A., Wang, J., 2002. Technical aspects and utility of fMRI using BOLD and ASL. *Clin Neurophysiol 113*, 621-634.

Dickerson, B.C., Goncharova, I., Sullivan, M.P., Forchetti, C., Wilson, R.S., Bennett, D.A., Beckett, L.A., deToledo-Morrell, L., 2001. MRI-derived entorhinal and hippocampal atrophy in incipient and very mild Alzheimer's disease. *Neurobiol Aging 22*, 747-754.

Dickerson, B.C., Salat, D.H., Bates, J.F., Atiya, M., Killiany, R.J., Greve, D.N., Dale, A.M., Stern, C.E., Blacker, D., Albert, M.S., Sperling, R.A., 2004. Medial temporal lobe function and structure in mild cognitive impairment. *Ann Neurol 56*, 27-35.

Dickerson, B.C., Salat, D.H., Greve, D.N., Chua, E.F., Rand-Giovannetti, E., Rentz, D.M., Bertram, L., Mullin, K., Tanzi, R.E., Blacker, D., Albert, M.S., Sperling, R.A., 2005. Increased hippocampal activation in mild cognitive impairment compared to normal aging and AD. *Neurology 65*, 404-411.

Dickson, D., 2003. Neurodegeneration: the molecular pathology of dementia and movement disorders, Blackwell Publishing.

Donnemiller, E., Heilmann, J., Wenning, G.K., Berger, W., Decristoforo, C., Moncayo, R., Poewe, W., Ransmayr, G., 1997. Brain perfusion scintigraphy with 99mTc-HMPAO or 99mTc-ECD and 123I-beta-CIT single-photon emission tomography in dementia of the Alzheimer-type and diffuse Lewy body disease. *Eur J Nucl Med 24*, 320-325.

Drzezga, A., Grimmer, T., Henriksen, G., Stangier, I., Perneczky, R., Diehl-Schmid, J., Mathis, C.A., Klunk, W.E., Price, J., Dekosky, S., Wester, H., Schwaiger, M., Kurz, A., 2008. Imaging of amyloid plaques and cerebral glucose metabolism in semantic dementia and Alzheimer's disease. *Neuroimage 39,* 619-633.

Drzezga, A., Grimmer, T., Riemenschneider, M., Lautenschlager, N., Siebner, H., Alexopoulus, P., Minoshima, S., Schwaiger, M., Kurz, A., 2005. Prediction of individual clinical outcome in MCI by means of genetic assessment and (18)F-FDG PET. *J Nucl Med 46,* 1625-1632.

Du, A., Schuff, N., Kramer, J.H., Rosen, H.J., Gorno-Tempini, M.L., Rankin, K., Miller, B.L., Weiner, M.W., 2007. Different regional patterns of cortical thinning in Alzheimer's disease and frontotemporal dementia. *Brain 130,* 1159-1166.

Du, A.T., Jahng, G.H., Hayasaka, S., Kramer, J.H., Rosen, H.J., Gorno-Tempini, M.L., Rankin, K.P., Miller, B.L., Weiner, M.W., Schuff, N., 2006. Hypoperfusion in frontotemporal dementia and Alzheimer disease by arterial spin labeling MRI. *Neurology 67,* 1215-1220.

Du, A.T., Schuff, N., Kramer, J.H., Ganzer, S., Zhu, X.P., Jagust, W.J., Miller, B.L., Reed, B.R., Mungas, D., Yaffe, K., Chui, H.C., Weiner, M.W., 2004. Higher atrophy rate of entorhinal cortex than hippocampus in AD. *Neurology 62,* 422-427.

Dubois, B., Feldman, H.H., Jacova, C., Dekosky, S.T., Barberger-Gateau, P., Cummings, J., Delacourte, A., Galasko, D., Gauthier, S., Jicha, G., Meguro, K., O'brien, J., Pasquier, F., Robert, P., Rossor, M., Salloway, S., Stern, Y., Visser, P.J., Scheltens, P., 2007. Research criteria for the diagnosis of Alzheimer's disease: revising the NINCDS-ADRDA criteria. *Lancet Neurol 6,* 734-746.

Eustache, F., Desgranges, B., Aupee, A., Guillery, B., Baron, J., 2000. Functional neuroanatomy of amnesia: positron emission tomography studies. *Microsc Res Tech 51,* 94-100.

Fellgiebel, A., Siessmeier, T., Scheurich, A., Winterer, G., Bartenstein, P., Schmidt, L.G., Müller, M.J., 2004. Association of elevated phospho-tau levels with Alzheimer-typical 18F-fluoro-2-deoxy-d-glucose positron emission tomography findings in patients with mild cognitive impairment. *Biol Psychiatry 56,* 279-283.

Fellgiebel, A., Wille, P., Müller, M.J., Winterer, G., Scheurich, A., Vucurevic, G., Schmidt, L.G., Stoeter, P., 2004. Ultrastructural hippocampal and white matter alterations in mild cognitive impairment: a diffusion tensor imaging study. *Dement Geriatr Cogn Disord 18,* 101-108.

Forsberg, A., Engler, H., Almkvist, O., Blomquist, G., Hagman, G., Wall, A., Ringheim, A., Långström, B., Nordberg, A., in press. PET imaging of amyloid deposition in patients with mild cognitive impairment. *Neurobiol Aging*.

Foster, N.L., Heidebrink, J.L., Clark, C.M., Jagust, W.J., Arnold, S.E., Barbas, N.R., DeCarli, C.S., Turner, R.S., Koeppe, R.A., Higdon, R., Minoshima, S., 2007. FDG-PET improves accuracy in distinguishing frontotemporal dementia and Alzheimer's disease. *Brain 130*, 2616-2635.

Fox, N.C., Jenkins, R., Leary, S.M., Stevenson, V.L., Losseff, N.A., Crum, W.R., Harvey, R.J., Rossor, M.N., Miller, D.H., Thompson, A.J., 2000. Progressive cerebral atrophy in MS: a serial study using registered, volumetric MRI. *Neurology 54*, 807-812.

Fox, N.C., Scahill, R.I., Crum, W.R., Rossor, M.N., 1999. Correlation between rates of brain atrophy and cognitive decline in AD. *Neurology 52*, 1687-1689.

Fox, N.C., Schott, J.M., 2004. Imaging cerebral atrophy: normal ageing to Alzheimer's disease. *Lancet 363*, 392-394.

Frisoni, G.B., 2001. Structural imaging in the clinical diagnosis of Alzheimer's disease: problems and tools. *J Neurol Neurosurg Psychiatry 70*, 711-718.

Garibotto, V., Borroni, B., Kalbe, E., Herholz, K., Salmon, E., Holtoff, V., Sorbi, S., Cappa, S., Padovani, A., Fazio, F., Perani, D., in press, Education and occupation as proxies for reserve in aMCI converters and AD: FDG-PET evidence. *Neurology*.

Gauthier, S., Reisberg, B., Zaudig, M., Petersen, R.C., Ritchie, K., Broich, K., Belleville, S., Brodaty, H., Bennett, D., Chertkow, H., Cummings, J.L., de Leon, M., Feldman, H., Ganguli, M., Hampel, H., Scheltens, P., Tierney, M.C., Whitehouse, P., Winblad, B., 2006. Mild cognitive impairment. *Lancet 367*, 1262-1270.

Gazzaley, A., Cooney, J.W., Rissman, J., D'Esposito, M., 2005. Top-down suppression deficit underlies working memory impairment in normal aging. *Nat Neurosci 8*, 1298-1300.

Gold, G., Giannakopoulos, P., Herrmann, F.R., Bouras, C., Kövari, E., 2007. Identification of Alzheimer and vascular lesion thresholds for mixed dementia. *Brain 130*, 2830-2836.

Goldman, W.P., Price, J.L., Storandt, M., Grant, E.A., McKeel, D.W.J., Rubin, E.H., Morris, J.C., 2001. Absence of cognitive impairment or decline in preclinical Alzheimer's disease. *Neurology 56*, 361-367.

Gorno-Tempini, M.L., Hutton, C., Josephs, O., Deichmann, R., Price, C., Turner, R., 2002. Echo time dependence of bold contrast and susceptibility artifacts. *Neuroimage 15*, 136-142.

Gunter, J.L., Shiung, M.M., Manduca, A., Jack, C.R.J., 2003. Methodological considerations for measuring rates of brain atrophy. *J Magn Reson Imaging 18*, 16-24.

Götz, J., Schild, A., Hoerndli, F., Pennanen, L., 2004. Amyloid-induced neurofibrillary tangle formation in alzheimerAlzheimer's disease: insight from transgenic mouse and tissue-culture models. *Int J Dev Neurosci 22*, 453-465.

Halldin, C., Gulyás, B., Farde, L., 2001. PET studies with carbon-11 radioligands in neuropsychopharmacological drug development. *Curr Pharm Des 7*, 1907-1929.

Hansen, L.A., Masliah, E., Galasko, D., Terry, R.D., 1993. Plaque-only Alzheimer disease is usually the Lewy body variant, and vice versa. *J Neuropathol Exp Neurol 52*, 648-654.

Harris, G.J., Lewis, R.F., Satlin, A., English, C.D., Scott, T.M., Yurgelun-Todd, D.A., Renshaw, P.F., 1996. Dynamic susceptibility contrast MRI of regional cerebral blood volume in Alzheimer's disease. *Am J Psychiatry 153*, 721-724.

Haxby, J.V., Grady, C.L., Koss, E., Horwitz, B., Schapiro, M., Friedland, R.P., Rapoport, S.I., 1988. Heterogeneous anterior-posterior metabolic patterns in dementia of the Alzheimer type. *Neurology 38*, 1853-1863.

Head, D., Buckner, R.L., Shimony, J.S., Williams, L.E., Akbudak, E., Conturo, T.E., McAvoy, M., Morris, J.C., Snyder, A.Z., 2004. Differential vulnerability of anterior white matter in nondemented aging with minimal acceleration in dementia of the Alzheimer type: evidence from diffusion tensor imaging. *Cereb Cortex 14*, 410-423.

Herholz, K., 2003. PET studies in dementia. *Ann Nucl Med 17*, 79-89.

Herholz, K., Nordberg, A., Salmon, E., Perani, D., Kessler, J., Mielke, R., Halber, M., Jelic, V., Almkvist, O., Collette, F., Alberoni, M., Kennedy, A., Hasselbalch, S., Fazio, F., Heiss, W.D., 1999. Impairment of neocortical metabolism predicts progression in Alzheimer's disease. *Dement Geriatr Cogn Disord 10*, 494-504.

Herholz, K., Perani, D., Salmon, E., Franck, G., Fazio, F., Heiss, W.D., Comar, D., 1993. Comparability of FDG PET studies in probable Alzheimer's disease. *J Nucl Med 34*, 1460-1466.

Herholz, K., Salmon, E., Perani, D., Baron, J.C., Holthoff, V., Frölich, L., Schönknecht, P., Ito, K., Mielke, R., Kalbe, E., Zündorf, G., Delbeuck, X., Pelati, O., Anchisi, D., Fazio, F., Kerrouche, N., Desgranges, B., Eustache, F., Beuthien-Baumann, B., Menzel, C., 2002. Discrimination between Alzheimer dementia and controls by automated analysis of multicenter FDG PET. *Neuroimage 17*, 302-316.

Herholz, K., Weisenbach, S., Kalbe, E., Diederich, N.J., Heiss, W., 2005. Cerebral acetylcholine esterase activity in mild cognitive impairment. *Neuroreport 16*, 1431-1434.

Herholz, K., Weisenbach, S., Zündorf, G., Lenz, O., Schröder, H., Bauer, B., Kalbe, E., Heiss, W., 2004. In vivo study of acetylcholine esterase in basal forebrain, amygdala, and cortex in mild to moderate Alzheimer disease. *Neuroimage 21*, 136-143.

Hisanaga, K., Suzuki, H., Tanji, H., Mochizuki, H., Iwasaki, Y., Sato, N., Jin, K., 2001. Fluoro-dopa and FDG positron emission tomography in a case of pathologically verified pure diffuse Lewy body disease. *J Neurol 248*, 905-906.

Hoffman, J.M., Welsh-Bohmer, K.A., Hanson, M., Crain, B., Hulette, C., Earl, N., Coleman, R.E., 2000. FDG PET imaging in patients with pathologically verified dementia. *J Nucl Med 41*, 1920-1928.

Hu, X.S., Okamura, N., Arai, H., Higuchi, M., Matsui, T., Tashiro, M., Shinkawa, M., Itoh, M., Ido, T., Sasaki, H., 2000. 18F-fluorodopa PET study of striatal dopamine uptake in the diagnosis of dementia with Lewy bodies. *Neurology 55*, 1575-1577.

Ince, P., 2001. Dementia with Lewy bodies. *Adv Exp Med Biol 487*, 135-145.

Irizarry, M.C., Hyman, B.T., 2001. Alzheimer disease therapeutics. *J Neuropathol Exp Neurol 60*, 923-928.

Ishii, K., Sasaki, M., Yamaji, S., Sakamoto, S., Kitagaki, H., Mori, E., 1998. Relatively preserved hippocampal glucose metabolism in mild Alzheimer's disease. *Dement Geriatr Cogn Disord 9*, 317-322.

Ishii, K., Soma, T., Kono, A.K., Sofue, K., Miyamoto, N., Yoshikawa, T., Mori, E., Murase, K., 2007. Comparison of regional brain volume and glucose metabolism between patients with mild dementia with Lewy bodies and those with mild Alzheimer's disease. *J Nucl Med 48*, 704-711.

Iyo, M., Namba, H., Fukushi, K., Shinotoh, H., Nagatsuka, S., Suhara, T., Sudo, Y., Suzuki, K., Irie, T., 1997. Measurement of acetylcholinesterase by positron emission tomography in the brains of healthy controls and patients with Alzheimer's disease. *Lancet 349*, 1805-1809.

Jack, C.R.J., Dickson, D.W., Parisi, J.E., Xu, Y.C., Cha, R.H., O'Brien, P.C., Edland, S.D., Smith, G.E., Boeve, B.F., Tangalos, E.G., Kokmen, E., Petersen, R.C., 2002. Antemortem MRI findings correlate with hippocampal neuropathology in typical aging and dementia. *Neurology 58*, 750-757.

Jack, C.R.J., Shiung, M.M., Gunter, J.L., O'Brien, P.C., Weigand, S.D., Knopman, D.S., Boeve, B.F., Ivnik, R.J., Smith, G.E., Cha, R.H., Tangalos, E.G., Petersen, R.C., 2004. Comparison of different MRI brain atrophy rate measures with clinical disease progression in AD. *Neurology 62*, 591-600.

Jagust, W., Thisted, R., Devous, M.D.S., Van Heertum, R., Mayberg, H., Jobst, K., Smith, A.D., Borys, N., 2001. Spect perfusion imaging in the diagnosis of Alzheimer's disease: a clinical-pathologic study. *Neurology 56*, 950-956.

Johnson, N.A., Jahng, G., Weiner, M.W., Miller, B.L., Chui, H.C., Jagust, W.J., Gorno-Tempini, M.L., Schuff, N., 2005. Pattern of cerebral hypoperfusion in Alzheimer disease and mild cognitive impairment measured with arterial spin-labeling mr imaging: initial experience. *Radiology 234*, 851-859.

Kantarci, K., Jack, C.R.J., Xu, Y.C., Campeau, N.G., O'Brien, P.C., Smith, G.E., Ivnik, R.J., Boeve, B.F., Kokmen, E., Tangalos, E.G., Petersen, R.C., 2001. Mild cognitive impairment and Alzheimer disease: regional diffusivity of water. *Radiology 219*, 101-107.

Kantarci, K., Petersen, R.C., Boeve, B.F., Knopman, D.S., Weigand, S.D., O'Brien, P.C., Shiung, M.M., Smith, G.E., Ivnik, R.J., Tangalos, E.G., Jack, C.R.J., 2005. Dwi predicts future progression to Alzheimer disease in amnestic mild cognitive impairment. *Neurology 64*, 902-904.

Karas, G.B., Scheltens, P., Rombouts, S.A.R.B., Visser, P.J., van Schijndel, R.A., Fox, N.C., Barkhof, F., 2004. Global and local gray matter loss in mild cognitive impairment and Alzheimer's disease. *Neuroimage 23*, 708-716.

Katzman, R., Fox, P., 1999. The world-wide impact of dementia. projections of prevalence and costs. In Mayeaux, R., Christen, Y., (Eds.), *Epidemiology of Alzheimer's disease: from gene to prevention.* Springer-Verlag, 1-17.

Kawas, C.H., 2003. Clinical practice. early Alzheimer's disease. *N Engl J Med 349*, 1056-1063.

Kemppainen, N., Ruottinen, H., Nâgren, K., Rinne, J.O., 2000. PET shows that striatal dopamine D1 and D2 receptors are differentially affected in AD. *Neurology 55*, 205-209.

Kepe, V., Huang, S., Small, G.W., Satyamurthy, N., Barrio, J.R., 2006. Visualizing pathology deposits in the living brain of patients with Alzheimer's disease. *Methods Enzymol 412*, 144-160.

Kerrouche, N., Herholz, K., Mielke, R., Holthoff, V., Baron, J., 2006. 18FDG PET in vascular dementia: differentiation from Alzheimer's disease using voxel-based multivariate analysis. *J Cereb Blood Flow Metab 26*, 1213-1221.

Kippenhan, J.S., Barker, W.W., Nagel, J., Grady, C., Duara, R., 1994. Neural-network classification of normal and Alzheimer's disease subjects using high-resolution and low-resolution PET cameras. *J Nucl Med 35*, 7-15.

Kipps, C.M., Duggins, A.J., Mahant, N., Gomes, L., Ashburner, J., McCusker, E.A., 2005. Progression of structural neuropathology in preclinical huntington's disease: a tensor based morphometry study. *J Neurol Neurosurg Psychiatry 76*, 650-655.

Klunk, W.E., Engler, H., Nordberg, A., Wang, Y., Blomqvist, G., Holt, D.P., Bergström, M., Savitcheva, I., Huang, G., Estrada, S., Ausén, B., Debnath, M.L., Barletta, J., Price, J.C., Sandell, J., Lopresti, B.J., Wall, A., Koivisto, P., Antoni, G., Mathis, C.A., 2004. Imaging brain amyloid in Alzheimer's disease with pittsburgh compound-B. *Ann Neurol 55*, 306-319.

Knopman, D.S., 2006. Current treatment of mild cognitive impairment and Alzheimer's disease. *Curr Neurol Neurosci Rep 6*, 365-371.

Knopman, D.S., DeKosky, S.T., Cummings, J.L., Chui, H., Corey-Bloom, J., Relkin, N., Small, G.W., Miller, B., Stevens, J.C., 2001. Practice parameter: diagnosis of dementia (an evidence-based review). Report of the quality standards subcommittee of the American Academy of Neurology. *Neurology 56*, 1143-1153.

Kuhl, D.E., Minoshima, S., Frey, K.A., Foster, N.L., Kilbourn, M.R., Koeppe, R.A., 2000. Limited donepezil inhibition of acetylcholinesterase measured with positron emission tomography in living Alzheimer cerebral cortex. *Ann Neurol 48*, 391-395.

de Leon, M., Mosconi, L., Blennow, K., DeSanti, S., Zinkowski, R., Mehta, P., Pratico, D., et al., 2007. Imaging and csf studies in the preclinical diagnosis of Alzheimer's disease. *Ann N Y Acad Sci 1097*, 114-145.

Leow, A.D., Yanovsky, I., Chiang, M., Lee, A.D., Klunder, A.D., Lu, A., Becker, J.T., Davis, S.W., Toga, A.W., Thompson, P.M., 2007. Statistical properties of jacobian maps and the realization of unbiased large-deformation nonlinear image registration. *IEEE Trans Med Imaging 26*, 822-832.

Liu, Y., Stern, Y., Chun, M.R., Jacobs, D.M., Yau, P., Goldman, J.E., 1997. Pathological correlates of extrapyramidal signs in Alzheimer's disease. *Ann Neurol 41*, 368-374.

Logothetis, N.K., Pauls, J., Augath, M., Trinath, T., Oeltermann, A., 2001. Neurophysiological investigation of the basis of the fMRI signal. *Nature 412*, 150-157.

Logothetis, N.K., Pfeuffer, J., 2004. On the nature of the bold fMRI contrast mechanism. *Magn Reson Imaging 22*, 1517-1531.

Logothetis, N.K., Wandell, B.A., 2004. Interpreting the bold signal. *Annu Rev Physiol 66*, 735-769.

Machulda, M.M., Ward, H.A., Borowski, B., Gunter, J.L., Cha, R.H., O'Brien, P.C., Petersen, R.C., Boeve, B.F., Knopman, D., Tang-Wai, D.F., Ivnik, R.J., Smith, G.E., Tangalos, E.G., Jack, C.R.J., 2003. Comparison of memory fMRI response among normal, MCI, and Alzheimer's patients. *Neurology 61*, 500-506.

Maetzler, W., Reimold, M., Liepelt, I., Solbach, C., Leyhe, T., Schweitzer, K., Eschweiler, G.W., Mittelbronn, M., Gaenslen, A., Uebele, M., Reischl, G., Gasser, T., Machulla, H., Bares, R., Berg, D., 2007. [(11)C]PIB binding in Parkinson's disease dementia. *Neuroimage 39,* 1027-1033 .

Mayeux, R., Sano, M., 1999. Treatment of Alzheimer's disease. *N Engl J Med 341*, 1670-1679.

McDowell, I., Xi, G., Lindsay, J., Tierney, M., 2007. Mapping the connections between education and dementia. *J Clin Exp Neuropsychol 29*, 127-141.

McKeith, I., O'Brien, J., Walker, Z., Tatsch, K., Booij, J., Darcourt, J., Padovani, A., Giubbini, R., Bonuccelli, U., Volterrani, D., Holmes, C., Kemp, P., Tabet, N., Meyer, I., Reininger, C., 2007. Sensitivity and specificity of dopamine transporter imaging with 123I-FP-CIT SPECT in dementia with Lewy bodies: a phase III, multicentre study. *Lancet Neurol 6*, 305-313.

McKeith, I.G., Dickson, D.W., Lowe, J., Emre, M., O'Brien, J.T., Feldman, H., Cummings, J., Duda, J.E., Lippa, C., Perry, E.K., Aarsland, D., Arai, H., Ballard, C.G., Boeve, B., Burn, D.J., Costa, D., Del Ser, T., Dubois, B., Galasko, D., Gauthier, S., 2005. Diagnosis and management of dementia with Lewy bodies: third report of the DLB consortium. *Neurology 65*, 1863-1872.

McKeith, I.G., Galasko, D., Kosaka, K., Perry, E.K., Dickson, D.W., Hansen, L.A., Salmon, D.P., Lowe, J., Mirra, S.S., Byrne, E.J., Lennox, G., Quinn, N.P., Edwardson, J.A., Ince, P.G., Bergeron, C., Burns, A., Miller, B.L., Lovestone, S., Collerton, D., Jansen, E.N., 1996. Consensus guidelines for the clinical and pathologic diagnosis of dementia with Lewy bodies (DLB): report of the consortium on DLB international workshop. *Neurology 47*, 1113-1124.

McNeill, R., Sare, G.M., Manoharan, M., Testa, H.J., Mann, D.M.A., Neary, D., Snowden, J.S., Varma, A.R., 2007. Accuracy of single-photon emission computed tomography in differentiating frontotemporal dementia from Alzheimer's disease. *J Neurol Neurosurg Psychiatry 78*, 350-355.

Mega, M.S., Chu, T., Mazziotta, J.C., Trivedi, K.H., Thompson, P.M., Shah, A., Cole, G., Frautschy, S.A., Toga, A.W., 1999. Mapping biochemistry to metabolism: FDG-PET and amyloid burden in Alzheimer's disease. *Neuroreport 10*, 2911-2917.

Mielke, R., Herholz, K., Grond, M., Kessler, J., Heiss, W.D., 1994. Clinical deterioration in probable Alzheimer's disease correlates with progressive metabolic impairment of association areas. *Dementia 5*, 36-41.

Minoshima, S., Foster, N.L., Sima, A.A., Frey, K.A., Albin, R.L., Kuhl, D.E., 2001. Alzheimer's disease versus dementia with Lewy bodies: cerebral metabolic distinction with autopsy confirmation. *Ann Neurol 50*, 358-365.

Minoshima, S., Frey, K.A., Cross, D.J., Kuhl, D.E., 2004. Neurochemical imaging of dementias. *Semin Nucl Med 34*, 70-82.

Minoshima, S., Giordani, B., Berent, S., Frey, K.A., Foster, N.L., Kuhl, D.E., 1997. Metabolic reduction in the posterior cingulate cortex in very early Alzheimer's disease. *Ann Neurol 42*, 85-94.

Moeller, J.R., Ishikawa, T., Dhawan, V., Spetsieris, P., Mandel, F., Alexander, G.E., Grady, C., Pietrini, P., Eidelberg, D., 1996. The metabolic topography of normal aging. *J Cereb Blood Flow Metab 16*, 385-398.

Morris, R., Mucke, L., 2006. Alzheimer's disease: a needle from the haystack. *Nature 440*, 284-285.

Mosconi, L., 2005. Brain glucose metabolism in the early and specific diagnosis of Alzheimer's disease. FDG-PET studies in MCI and AD. *Eur J Nucl Med Mol Imaging 32*, 486-510.

Mosconi, L., Perani, D., Sorbi, S., Herholz, K., Nacmias, B., Holthoff, V., Salmon, E., Baron, J., De Cristofaro, M.T.R., Padovani, A., Borroni, B., Franceschi, M., Bracco, L., Pupi, A., 2004. MCI conversion to dementia and the ApoE genotype: a prediction study with FDG-PET. *Neurology 63*, 2332-2340.

Mosconi, L., Pupi, A., De Cristofaro, M.T.R., Fayyaz, M., Sorbi, S., Herholz, K., 2004. Functional interactions of the entorhinal cortex: an 18F-FDG PET study on normal aging and Alzheimer's disease. *J Nucl Med 45*, 382-392.

Mosconi, L., Tsui, W., De Santi, S., Li, J., Rusinek, H., Convit, A., Li, Y., Boppana, M., de Leon, M.J., 2005. Reduced hippocampal metabolism in

MCI and ad: automated FDG-PET image analysis. *Neurology 64*, 1860-1867.

Mudher, A., Lovestone, S., 2002. Alzheimer's disease-do tauists and baptists finally shake hands? *Trends Neurosci 25*, 22-26.

Mueller, S.G., Weiner, M.W., Thal, L.J., Petersen, R.C., Jack, C., Jagust, W., Trojanowski, J.Q., Toga, A.W., Beckett, L., 2005. The Alzheimer's disease neuroimaging initiative. *Neuroimaging Clin N Am 15*, 869-77, XI-XII.

Müller, M.J., Greverus, D., Weibrich, C., Dellani, P.R., Scheurich, A., Stoeter, P., Fellgiebel, A., 2007. Diagnostic utility of hippocampal size and mean diffusivity in amnestic MCI. *Neurobiol Aging 28*, 398-403.

Ngandu, T., von Strauss, E., Helkala, E., Winblad, B., Nissinen, A., Tuomilehto, J., Soininen, H., Kivipelto, M., 2007. Education and dementia: what lies behind the association? *Neurology 69*, 1442-1450.

Nordberg, A., 2004. PET imaging of amyloid in Alzheimer's disease. *Lancet Neurol 3*, 519-527.

Ogawa, S., Lee, T.M., Kay, A.R., Tank, D.W., 1990. Brain magnetic resonance imaging with contrast dependent on blood oxygenation. *Proc Natl Acad Sci U S A 87*, 9868-9872.

Padovani, A., Borroni, B., Brambati, S.M., Agosti, C., Broli, M., Alonso, R., Scifo, P., Bellelli, G., Alberici, A., Gasparotti, R., Perani, D., 2006. Diffusion tensor imaging and voxel based morphometry study in early progressive supranuclear palsy. *J Neurol Neurosurg Psychiatry 77*, 457-463.

Pasquier, J., Michel, B.F., Brenot-Rossi, I., Hassan-Sebbag, N., Sauvan, R., Gastaut, J.L., 2002. Value of (99m)Tc-ECD SPET for the diagnosis of dementia with Lewy bodies. *Eur J Nucl Med Mol Imaging 29*, 1342-1348.

Perneczky, R., Drzezga, A., Diehl-Schmid, J., Schmid, G., Wohlschläger, A., Kars, S., Grimmer, T., Wagenpfeil, S., Monsch, A., Kurz, A., 2006. Schooling mediates brain reserve in Alzheimer's disease: findings of fluoro-deoxy-glucose-positron emission tomography. *J Neurol Neurosurg Psychiatry 77*, 1060-1063.

Persson, J., Lind, J., Larsson, A., Ingvar, M., Cruts, M., Van Broeckhoven, C., Adolfsson, R., Nilsson, L., Nyberg, L., 2006. Altered brain white matter integrity in healthy carriers of the ApoE epsilon4 allele: a risk for AD? *Neurology 66*, 1029-1033.

Persson, J., Nyberg, L., Lind, J., Larsson, A., Nilsson, L., Ingvar, M., Buckner, R.L., 2006. Structure-function correlates of cognitive decline in aging. *Cereb Cortex 16*, 907-915.

Petersen, R.C., 2004. Mild cognitive impairment as a diagnostic entity. *J Intern Med 256*, 183-194.

Petersen, R.C., Doody, R., Kurz, A., Mohs, R.C., Morris, J.C., Rabins, P.V., Ritchie, K., Rossor, M., Thal, L., Winblad, B., 2001. Current concepts in mild cognitive impairment. *Arch Neurol 58*, 1985-1992.

Petit-Taboué, M.C., Landeau, B., Desson, J.F., Desgranges, B., Baron, J.C., 1998. Effects of healthy aging on the regional cerebral metabolic rate of glucose assessed with statistical parametric mapping. *Neuroimage 7*, 176-184.

Pike, K.E., Savage, G., Villemagne, V.L., Ng, S., Moss, S.A., Maruff, P., Mathis, C.A., Klunk, W.E., Masters, C.L., Rowe, C.C., 2007. Beta-amyloid imaging and memory in non-demented individuals: evidence for preclinical Alzheimer's disease. *Brain 130*, 2837-44. .

Pizzolato, G., Chierichetti, F., Fabbri, M., Cagnin, A., Dam, M., Ferlin, G., Battistin, L., 1996. Reduced striatal dopamine receptors in Alzheimer's disease: single photon emission tomography study with the d2 tracer [123I]-IBZM. *Neurology 47*, 1065-1068.

Praticò, D., Clark, C.M., Liun, F., Rokach, J., Lee, V.Y., Trojanowski, J.Q., 2002. Increase of brain oxidative stress in mild cognitive impairment: a possible predictor of Alzheimer disease. *Arch Neurol 59*, 972-976.

Rabinovici, G.D., Seeley, W.W., Kim, E.J., Gorno-Tempini, M.L., Rascovsky, K., Pagliaro, T.A., Allison, S.C., Halabi, C., Kramer, J.H., Johnson, J.K., Weiner, M.W., Forman, M.S., Trojanowski, J.Q., Dearmond, S.J., Miller, B.L., Rosen, H.J., 2007. Distinct MRI atrophy patterns in autopsy-proven Alzheimer's disease and frontotemporal lobar degeneration. *Am J Alzheimers Dis Other Demen 22*, 474-488.

Rajah, M.N., D'Esposito, M., 2005. Region-specific changes in prefrontal function with age: a review of PET and fMRI studies on working and episodic memory. *Brain 128*, 1964-1983.

Ransmayr, G., Seppi, K., Donnemiller, E., Luginger, E., Marksteiner, J., Riccabona, G., Poewe, W., Wenning, G.K., 2001. Striatal dopamine transporter function in dementia with Lewy bodies and Parkinson's disease. *Eur J Nucl Med 28*, 1523-1528.

Reiman, E.M., Caselli, R.J., Chen, K., Alexander, G.E., Bandy, D., Frost, J., 2001. Declining brain activity in cognitively normal apolipoprotein e epsilon 4 heterozygotes: a foundation for using positron emission tomography to efficiently test treatments to prevent Alzheimer's disease. *Proc Natl Acad Sci U S A 98*, 3334-3339.

Reiman, E.M., Caselli, R.J., Yun, L.S., Chen, K., Bandy, D., Minoshima, S., Thibodeau, S.N., Osborne, D., 1996. Preclinical evidence of Alzheimer's disease in persons homozygous for the epsilon 4 allele for apolipoprotein E. *N Engl J Med 334*, 752-758.

Reiman, E.M., Chen, K., Alexander, G.E., Caselli, R.J., Bandy, D., Osborne, D., Saunders, A.M., Hardy, J., 2004. Functional brain abnormalities in young adults at genetic risk for late-onset Alzheimer's dementia. *Proc Natl Acad Sci U S A 101*, 284-289.

Resnick, S.M., Pham, D.L., Kraut, M.A., Zonderman, A.B., Davatzikos, C., 2003. Longitudinal magnetic resonance imaging studies of older adults: a shrinking brain. *J Neurosci 23*, 3295-3301.

Rinne, J.O., Kaasinen, V., Järvenpää, T., Någren, K., Roivainen, A., Yu, M., Oikonen, V., Kurki, T., 2003. Brain acetylcholinesterase activity in mild cognitive impairment and early Alzheimer's disease. *J Neurol Neurosurg Psychiatry 74*, 113-115.

Rinne, J.O., Sahlberg, N., Ruottinen, H., Någren, K., Lehikoinen, P., 1998. Striatal uptake of the dopamine reuptake ligand [11C]beta-CFT is reduced in Alzheimer's disease assessed by positron emission tomography. *Neurology 50*, 152-156.

Roe, C.M., Xiong, C., Miller, J.P., Morris, J.C., 2007. Education and Alzheimer disease without dementia: support for the cognitive reserve hypothesis. *Neurology 68*, 223-228.

Rose, S.E., McMahon, K.L., Janke, A.L., O'Dowd, B., de Zubicaray, G., Strudwick, M.W., Chalk, J.B., 2006. Diffusion indices on magnetic resonance imaging and neuropsychological performance in amnestic mild cognitive impairment. *J Neurol Neurosurg Psychiatry 77*, 1122-1128.

Rypma, B., D'Esposito, M., 2000. Isolating the neural mechanisms of age-related changes in human working memory. *Nat Neurosci 3*, 509-515.

Salat, D.H., Tuch, D.S., Greve, D.N., van der Kouwe, A.J.W., Hevelone, N.D., Zaleta, A.K., Rosen, B.R., Fischl, B., Corkin, S., Rosas, H.D., Dale, A.M., 2005. Age-related alterations in white matter microstructure measured by diffusion tensor imaging. *Neurobiol Aging 26*, 1215-1227.

Scarmeas, N., Albert, S.M., Manly, J.J., Stern, Y., 2006. Education and rates of cognitive decline in incident Alzheimer's disease. *J Neurol Neurosurg Psychiatry 77*, 308-316.

Shinotoh, H., Aotsuka, A., Fukushi, K., Nagatsuka, S., Tanaka, N., Ota, T., Tanada, S., Irie, T., 2001. Effect of donepezil on brain acetylcholinesterase activity in patients with AD measured by PET. *Neurology 56*, 408-410.

Shinotoh, H., Namba, H., Fukushi, K., Nagatsuka, S., Tanaka, N., Aotsuka, A., Ota, T., Tanada, S., Irie, T., 2000. Progressive loss of cortical acetylcholinesterase activity in association with cognitive decline in Alzheimer's disease: a positron emission tomography study. *Ann Neurol 48*, 194-200.

Shoghi-Jadid, K., Small, G.W., Agdeppa, E.D., Kepe, V., Ercoli, L.M., Siddarth, P., Read, S., Satyamurthy, N., Petric, A., Huang, S., Barrio, J.R., 2002. Localization of neurofibrillary tangles and beta-amyloid plaques in the brains of living patients with Alzheimer disease. *Am J Geriatr Psychiatry 10*, 24-35.

Signorini, M., Paulesu, E., Friston, K., Perani, D., Colleluori, A., Lucignani, G., Grassi, F., Bettinardi, V., Frackowiak, R.S., Fazio, F., 1999. Rapid assessment of regional cerebral metabolic abnormalities in single subjects with quantitative and nonquantitative [18F]FDG PET: a clinical validation of statistical parametric mapping. *Neuroimage 9*, 63-80.

Silbert, L.C., Quinn, J.F., Moore, M.M., Corbridge, E., Ball, M.J., Murdoch, G., Sexton, G., Kaye, J.A., 2003. Changes in premorbid brain volume predict Alzheimer's disease pathology. *Neurology 61*, 487-492.

Singh, V., Chertkow, H., Lerch, J.P., Evans, A.C., Dorr, A.E., Kabani, N.J., 2006. Spatial patterns of cortical thinning in mild cognitive impairment and Alzheimer's disease. *Brain 129*, 2885-2893.

Small, G.W., Ercoli, L.M., Silverman, D.H., Huang, S.C., Komo, S., Bookheimer, S.Y., Lavretsky, H., Miller, K., Siddarth, P., Rasgon, N.L., Mazziotta, J.C., Saxena, S., Wu, H.M., Mega, M.S., Cummings, J.L., Saunders, A.M., Pericak-Vance, M.A., Roses, A.D., Barrio, J.R., Phelps, M.E., 2000. Cerebral metabolic and cognitive decline in persons at genetic risk for Alzheimer's disease. *Proc Natl Acad Sci U S A 97*, 6037-6042.

Small, G.W., Kepe, V., Ercoli, L.M., Siddarth, P., Bookheimer, S.Y., Miller, K.J., Lavretsky, H., Burggren, A.C., Cole, G.M., Vinters, H.V., Thompson, P.M., Huang, S., Satyamurthy, N., Phelps, M.E., Barrio, J.R., 2006. PET of brain amyloid and tau in mild cognitive impairment. *N Engl J Med 355*, 2652-2663.

Small, S.A., Perera, G.M., DeLaPaz, R., Mayeux, R., Stern, Y., 1999. Differential regional dysfunction of the hippocampal formation among elderly with memory decline and Alzheimer's disease. *Ann Neurol 45*, 466-472.

Smith, G.S., de Leon, M.J., George, A.E., Kluger, A., Volkow, N.D., McRae, T., Golomb, J., Ferris, S.H., Reisberg, B., Ciaravino, J., et al., 1992. Topography of cross-sectional and longitudinal glucose metabolic deficits in Alzheimer's disease. pathophysiologic implications. *Arch Neurol 49*, 1142-1150.

Snowdon, D.A., Ostwald, S.K., Kane, R.L., 1989. Education, survival, and independence in elderly catholic sisters, 1936-1988. *Am J Epidemiol 130*, 999-1012.

Soto, C., 2003. Unfolding the role of protein misfolding in neurodegenerative diseases. *Nat Rev Neurosci 4*, 49-60.

Stern, Y., 2002. What is cognitive reserve? theory and research application of the reserve concept. *J Int Neuropsychol Soc 8*, 448-460.

Stern, Y., Alexander, G.E., Prohovnik, I., Mayeux, R., 1992. Inverse relationship between education and parietotemporal perfusion deficit in Alzheimer's disease. *Ann Neurol 32*, 371-375.

Sullivan, E.V., Adalsteinsson, E., Pfefferbaum, A., 2006. Selective age-related degradation of anterior callosal fiber bundles quantified in vivo with fiber tracking. *Cereb Cortex 16*, 1030-1039.

Talbot, P.R., Lloyd, J.J., Snowden, J.S., Neary, D., Testa, H.J., 1998. A clinical role for 99mTc-HMPAO SPECT in the investigation of dementia? *J Neurol Neurosurg Psychiatry 64*, 306-313.

Tam, C.W.C., Burton, E.J., McKeith, I.G., Burn, D.J., O'Brien, J.T., 2005. Temporal lobe atrophy on MRI in Parkinson disease with dementia: a comparison with Alzheimer disease and dementia with Lewy bodies. *Neurology 64*, 861-865.

Taoka, T., Iwasaki, S., Sakamoto, M., Nakagawa, H., Fukusumi, A., Myochin, K., Hirohashi, S., Hoshida, T., Kichikawa, K., 2006. Diffusion anisotropy and diffusivity of white matter tracts within the temporal stem in Alzheimer disease: evaluation of the "tract of interest" by diffusion tensor tractography. *AJNR Am J Neuroradiol 27*, 1040-1045.

Taylor, J.P., Hardy, J., Fischbeck, K.H., 2002. Toxic proteins in neurodegenerative disease. *Science 296*, 1991-1995.

Thal, L.J., Kantarci, K., Reiman, E.M., Klunk, W.E., Weiner, M.W., Zetterberg, H., Galasko, D., Praticò, D., Griffin, S., Schenk, D., Siemers, E., 2006. The role of biomarkers in clinical trials for Alzheimer disease. *Alzheimer Dis Assoc Disord 20*, 6-15.

The Ronald and Nancy Reagan Research Institute of the Alzheimer's Association and, N.I.O.A.W.G., 1998. Consensus report of the working group on: "Molecular and biochemical markers of Alzheimer's disease". The Ronald and Nancy Reagan research institute of the Alzheimer's association and the national institute on aging working group. *Neurobiology of Aging 19*, 109-116.

Thompson, P.M., Hayashi, K.M., Dutton, R.A., Chiang, M., Leow, A.D., Sowell, E.R., De Zubicaray, G., Becker, J.T., Lopez, O.L., Aizenstein, H.J., Toga, A.W., 2007. Tracking Alzheimer's disease. *Ann N Y Acad Sci 1097*, 183-214.

de Toledo-Morrell, L., Stoub, T.R., Bulgakova, M., Wilson, R.S., Bennett, D.A., Leurgans, S., Wuu, J., Turner, D.A., 2004. MRI-derived entorhinal volume is a good predictor of conversion from MCI to AD. *Neurobiol Aging 25*, 1197-1203.

Tyrrell, P.J., Sawle, G.V., Ibanez, V., Bloomfield, P.M., Leenders, K.L., Frackowiak, R.S., Rossor, M.N., 1990. Clinical and positron emission tomographic studies in the 'extrapyramidal syndrome' of dementia of the Alzheimer type. *Arch Neurol 47*, 1318-1323.

Valla, J., Berndt, J.D., Gonzalez-Lima, F., 2001. Energy hypometabolism in posterior cingulate cortex of Alzheimer's patients: superficial laminar cytochrome oxidase associated with disease duration. *J Neurosci 21*, 4923-4930.

Visser, P.J., Scheltens, P., Verhey, F.R., Schmand, B., Launer, L.J., Jolles, J., Jonker, C., 1999. Medial temporal lobe atrophy and memory dysfunction as predictors for dementia in subjects with mild cognitive impairment. *J Neurol 246*, 477-485.

Waldemar, G., Dubois, B., Emre, M., Georges, J., McKeith, I., Rossor, M., Scheltens, P., Tariska, P., Winblad, B., EFNS., 2007. Recommendations for the diagnosis and magagement of Alzheimer's disease and other disorders associated with dementia: efns guideline. *European Journal of Neurology 14*, e1-e26.

Walker, Z., Costa, D.C., Ince, P., McKeith, I.G., Katona, C.L., 1999. In-vivo demonstration of dopaminergic degeneration in dementia with Lewy bodies. *Lancet 354*, 646-647.

Walker, Z., Costa, D.C., Janssen, A.G., Walker, R.W., Livingstone, G., Katona, C.L., 1997. Dementia with Lewy bodies: a study of post-synaptic dopaminergic receptors with iodine-123 iodobenzamide single-photon emission tomography. *Eur J Nucl Med 24*, 609-614.

Walker, Z., Costa, D.C., Walker, R.W.H., Shaw, K., Gacinovic, S., Stevens, T., Livingston, G., Ince, P., McKeith, I.G., Katona, C.L.E., 2002. Differentiation of dementia with Lewy bodies from Alzheimer's disease using a dopaminergic presynaptic ligand. *J Neurol Neurosurg Psychiatry 73*, 134-140.

Whitwell, J.L., Jack, C.R.J., 2005. Comparisons between Alzheimer disease, frontotemporal lobar degeneration, and normal aging with brain mapping. *Top Magn Reson Imaging 16*, 409-425.

Winblad, B., Kilander, L., Eriksson, S., Minthon, L., Båtsman, S., Wetterholm, A., Jansson-Blixt, C., Haglund, A., 2006. Donepezil in patients with severe Alzheimer's disease: double-blind, parallel-group, placebo-controlled study. *Lancet 367*, 1057-1065.

Winblad, B., Palmer, K., Kivipelto, M., Jelic, V., Fratiglioni, L., Wahlund, L.O., Nordberg, A., Bäckman, L., Albert, M., Almkvist, O., Arai, H., Basun, H., Blennow, K., de Leon, M., DeCarli, C., Erkinjuntti, T., Giacobini, E., Graff, C., Hardy, J., Jack, C., Jorm, A., Ritchie, K., van Duijn, C., Visser, P., Petersen, R. C., 2004. Mild cognitive impairment-beyond controversies, towards a consensus: report of the international working group on mild cognitive impairment. *J Intern Med 256*, 240-246.

Yamaguchi, S., Meguro, K., Itoh, M., Hayasaka, C., Shimada, M., Yamazaki, H., Yamadori, A., 1997. Decreased cortical glucose metabolism correlates with hippocampal atrophy in Alzheimer's disease as shown by MRI and PET. *J Neurol Neurosurg Psychiatry 62*, 596-600.

Zamrini, E., De Santi, S., Tolar, M., 2004. Imaging is superior to cognitive testing for early diagnosis of Alzheimer's disease. *Neurobiol Aging 25*, 685-691.

Zuendorf, G., Kerrouche, N., Herholz, K., Baron, J., 2003. Efficient principal component analysis for multivariate 3D voxel-based mapping of brain functional imaging data sets as applied to FDG-PET and normal aging. *Hum Brain Mapp 18*, 13-21.

In: Alzheimer's Diagnosis   ISBN: 978-1-61209-846-3
Editor: Charles E. Ronson, pp. 227-243   ©2011 Nova Science Publishers, Inc.

Chapter IX

Cerebrospinal Fluid Biomarkers for Alzheimer's Disease

Eliana Venturelli*, Chiara Villa and Elio Scarpini

Dept. of Neurological Sciences, University of Milan, IRCCS Fondazione
Ospedale Maggiore Policlinico, Milan, Italy

Abstract

Alzheimer's disease (AD), Lewy-body disease (LBD) and Frontotemporal Dementia (FTD) are the major causes of memory impairment and dementia. As new therapeutic agents are under testing for the different diseases, there is an ultimate need for an early differential diagnosis. Biomarkers can serve as early diagnostic indicators or as markers of preclinical pathological changes. Therefore, diagnostic markers in the cerebrospinal fluid (CSF) have become a rapidly growing research field, since CSF is in direct contact with the central nervous system (CNS) and is supposed to reflect the brain environment.

So far, three CSF biomarkers, the 42 amino acid form of β-amyloid (Aβ), total tau and phosphotau, have been validated in a number of studies. These CSF markers have high sensitivity to differentiate early and incipient AD from normal aging, depression, alcohol dementia and

---

* Correspondence concerning this article should be addressed to: Eliana Venturelli, phone +390255033858; Fax: +390250320430; e-mail: eliana.venturelli@unimi.it.

Parkinson's disease, but lower specificity against other dementias, such as FTD and LBD.

This chapter reviews CSF biomarkers for AD, with emphasis on their role in the clinical diagnosis.

1. Introduction

Alzheimer's disease (AD) is the most common cause of dementia in the elderly, with a prevalence of 5% after 65 years of age, increasing to about 30% in people aged 85 years or older. The diagnosis of AD is currently based on the identification of dementia according to DSMIV (American Psychiatric Association, 1994) and specific clinical symptoms suggesting AD together with the exclusion of other causes of dementia as evaluated by laboratory tests and computerized tomography (CT) (NINCDS-ADRDA criteria; McKhann et al., 1984). AD is clinically characterized by progressive cognitive impairment, including impaired judgement, decision-making and orientation, often accompanied, in later stages, by psychobehavioural disturbances as well as language impairment. AD is associated with brain atrophy (Figure 1), with smaller hippocampal and amygdalar volumes at MRI.

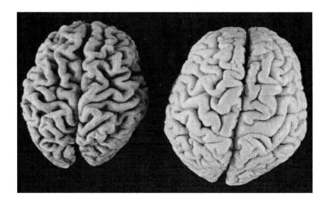

Figure 1. AD versus normal brain.

1.1. Pathogenesis of Alzheimer's Disease

The two major neuropathologic hallmarks of AD are extracellular Amyloid beta (Aβ) plaques and intracellular neurofibrillary tangles (NFTs)

(Figure 2). The production of Aβ, which represents a crucial step in AD pathogenesis, is the result of an aberrant cleavage of the Amyloiod peptide Precursor Protein (APP), that is overexpressed in AD (Griffin, 2006). Aβ forms highly insoluble and proteolysis resistant fibrils known as senile plaques (SP). In contrast to the low-fibrillar Aβ plaques (diffuse plaques), highly fibrillar (amyloidogenic) forms of Aβ plaques are associated with glial and neuritic changes of the surrounding tissue (neuritic-plaques) (Hoozemans et al., 2006). NFTs are composed of the tau protein. In healthy controls, tau is a component of microtubules, which represent the internal support structures for the transport of nutrients, vesicles, mitochondria and chromosomes within the cell. Microtubules also stabilize growing axons, which are necessary for the development and growth of neurites (Griffin, 2006). In AD, tau protein is abnormally hyperphosphorilated and forms insoluble fibrils, which originate deposits within the cell.

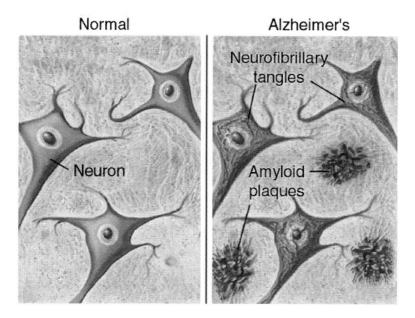

Figure 2. Schematic representation of the two major neuropathologic hallmarks of AD: extracellular Amyloid β (Aβ) plaques and intracellular neurofibrillary tangles (NFTs).

1.2. Biomarkers

In view of existing and emerging therapeutic compounds there is a great need for reliable biochemical diagnostic markers (biomarkers), allowing early and accurate diagnosis of dementia, particularly for AD. Cerebrospinal fluid (CSF) is in direct contact with the extracellular space of the brain, and thus biochemical changes in the brain are reflected in CSF. A diagnostic marker for AD should reflect a central pathogenic process of the disorder, such as the degeneration of neurons and their synapses and the defining lesions, naming, senile plaques, deriving from the aggregation of Aβ, and NFTs, resulting from hyperphosphorylation of tau protein. A clinically useful diagnostic marker should have a sensitivity exceeding 80% and a specificity above 80% according to the statement of the Consensus Group for Biomarkers (The Ronald and Nancy Regan Research Institute of the Alzheimer's Association, 1998). The goals of this declaration were to define characteristics of an ideal biological marker, to outline the process whereby a biological marker gains acceptance in the medical and scientific community and to review the current status of all proposed biomarkers for AD. According to the guidelines proposed, a diagnostic marker for AD should reflect a central pathogenic process of the disorder. It must have the following characteristics:

1. be able to detect a fundamental feature of Alzheimer's neuropathology
2. validated in neuropathologically confirmed AD cases
3. precise (able to detect AD early in its course and distinguish it from other dementias)
4. reliable
5. non-invasive
6. simple to perform
7. inexpensive.

Results on biomarkers must be replicated in at least two independent studies published in peer-review journals before being accepted by the scientific community.

In light of these considerations, at present suggested biomarkers for AD are total tau protein (T-tau), Aβ42, and phospho-tau (P-tau).

1.3. Mild Cognitive Impairment

Mild Cognitive Impairment (MCI) is an etiologically heterogeneous syndrome characterized by memory performances below normal levels (corrected for age). Despite this modest cognitive impairment, the global intellectual functioning is preserved as well as activities of daily living. A substantial proportion of patients with MCI later develop clinical AD (Petersen, 1995). During this preclinical period, there is a gradual loss of axons and neurons, and at a certain threshold the first symptoms, most often impaired episodic memory, appear (Hansson et al., 2006). At autopsy, subjects with MCI showed a broad spectrum of morphological brain changes, including typical AD pathological characteristics (Petersen et al., 1997). Therefore, MCI partly represents a predementia stage of AD. To maximise the benefits of therapeutic strategies that maintain cognitive and functional performances or delay the progression of the neurodegenerative process, it is essential to identify AD at the stage of MCI. Because the pattern of neuropsychological impairment in MCI is etiologically non-specific, biochemical and neuroimaging markers will be required to establish the diagnosis so early in the course of the disease. To date, CSF markers have been shown to have a high predictive power for identifying subjects with MCI who have the greatest risk of progressing to clinical AD (Riemenschneider et al., 2002).

2. Amyloid β (Aβ)

One of the first major findings in AD research was that Amyloid β (Aβ) is the main protein constituent of senile plaques (Masters et al., 1985). Aβ is produced continuously as a soluble protein during normal cellular metabolism and is secreted into the extracellular space and, thus, into the cerebrospinal fluid (CSF) (Seubert et al, 1992; Haass al., 1992). Aβ is a proteolytic cleavage product derived from the APP (Kang et al., 1987). The APP gene is located on chromosome 21 (St George-Hyslop et al., 1987), has three major alternate splicing variants with 770, 751 or 695 amino acids and is metabolized along two pathways. For the generation of Aβ, APP is cleaved after position 671 by a protease referred to as β-secretase, resulting in the release of a large N-terminal derivate called β-secretase-cleaved soluble APP (β-sAPP), and in a second step by the γ-secretase complex releasing free Aβ. The amyloid peptides comprise a heterogeneous set of N- and C-terminally truncated peptides. The three best known C-terminally truncated Aβ peptides are Aβ38, Aβ40 and Aβ42 (Schoonenboom et al., 2005). Aβ38 has been found to be the second prominent soluble Aβ peptide species in CSF after Aβ40 (Wiltfang et al., 2002) (Figure 3).

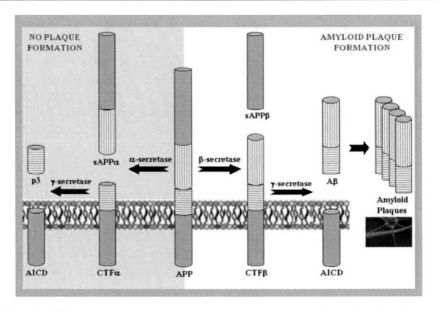

Figure 3. APP Processing: α-secretase and γ-secretase produce non-plaque forming p3, whereas β-secretase and γ-secretase produce amyloid plaque-forming Aβ. The different regions of the APP protein are indicated.

The role of APP in the central nervous system is not clear yet. A number of functional domains have been mapped to the extra- and intracellular region of APP, including metal (copper and zinc) binding motifs, extracellular matrix components (heparin, collagen and laminin), neurotrophic and adhesion domains. Thus far, a thropic role for APP has been suggested, as it stimulates neurite outgrowth in a variety of experimental settings. The N-terminal heparin-binding domain of APP also stimulates neurite outgrowth and promotes synaptogenesis. In addition, an "RHDS" motif near the extralumenal portion of APP likely promotes cell adhesion, possibly acting in an integrin-like manner. Similarly, APP colocalizes with integrins on the surface of axons at sites of adhesion (Storey et al., 1996, Yamazaki et al., 1997). Despite APP was initially proposed to act as a cell surface receptor, the evidence supporting this hypothesis has been unconvincing.

2.1. Aβ Levels in CSF

The discovery that the Aβ42 peptide precipitated in unsoluble aggregates forming senile plaques led to the development of ELISAs, specific for this peptide. At present, five different ELISA methods specific for Aβ42 exist. At least 20 studies have been conducted on a total of more than 2,000 patients and controls, showing a reduction of Aβ42 by about 50% in AD patients compared with non-demented controls of the same age (see Blennow and Hampel, 2003 for review). The reduction in CSF of AD patients may be due to Aβ42 deposition in senile plaques as an autopsy study has shown strong correlation between high numbers of plaques in the neocortex and hippocampus and low Aβ42 levels in ventricular CSF (Strozyk et al., 2003).

Moderately low levels were also found in Lewy Body Dementia (LBD; Kanemaru et al., 2000). A mild or moderate decrease in Aβ42 was found in a percentage of patients with Frontotemporal Dementia (FTD) and Vascular Dementia (VaD) (Sjögren et al., 2000), whereas normal Aβ42 were found in depression, Parkinson's disease and Progressive Supranuclear Palsy (PSP) (Holmberg et al., 2003).

CSF Aβ38 and Aβ40 levels were similar in patients with AD compared with control subjects. All three Aβ peptides were related to each other, with the strongest correlation between CSF Aβ38 and Aβ40 (Schoonenboom et al., 2005). The Aβ42/Aβ40 and Aβ42/Aβ38 ratios are considered to give information about the disease progression, typically in the early stage of disease, because the cerebral deposition of Aβ42 probably starts already before the disease becomes clinically overt (Blennow and Hampel, 2003). This observation is in agreement with an earlier report showing an increased Aβ42/Aβ40 ratio before the clinical onset of AD (Kanai et al., 1998). CSF Aβ42 alone is considered to be a stage marker, reflecting the presence of the disease at certain stage. It would be of interest to investigate the ratio of Aβ42 to Aβ40 and Aβ38 in a group of patients with mild cognitive impairment, observed longitudinally, to be informed when Aβ42 starts to decrease in CSF, as compared with Aβ38 and Aβ40, in relation with clinical progression.

3. Total Tau Protein (T-tau)

Tau is a normal brain phosphoprotein that promotes the assembly and stability of neuronal axons by binding to microtubules (Goedert, 1993). There are six different isoforms of tau in the human brain and numerous phosphorylation sites. In AD, hyperphosphorylated tau is the principal component of paired helical filaments (PHFs), which form neurofibrillary tangles, neurophil threads and senile plaque neuritis (Grundke-Iqbal et al.,

1986). These formations result in the disintegration of microtubules. Tau pathology can also be observed in other neurodegenerative disease, but it differs from AD patients at the molecular level (Hasegawa, 2006). Tau protein was quantified in the CSF under the hypothesis that it is released extracellularly as a result of the neurodegenerative process. CSF levels of total tau probably reflect the intensity of neuronal damage and degeneration (Andreasen et al., 1998).

3.1. Total Tau Levels in CSF

Three different ELISAs based on monoclonal antibodies that detect all isoforms of tau independent of the phosphorilation state of the protein have been developed measuring T-tau in CSF (Blennow et al., 1995). Using these ELISAs, a moderate to marked increase in T-tau in AD has consistently been demonstrated in more than 50 studies (Andreasen et al., 2003). CSF levels of T-tau probably reflect the intensity of neuronal damage and degeneration (Andreasen et al., 1998). High CFS levels are expected in all disorders with neuronal degeneration or damage. This has been confirmed in conditions such as Creutzfeldt-Jacob disease (Otto et al., 1997) and acute stroke (Hesse et al., 2000). Mild elevation of T-tau was also found in a proportion of cases with other dementias, such as FTD, LBD and VaD. In contrast, subjects with other neurological disorders, including Parkinson's disease and PSP, or psychiatric disorders (e.g. depression) showed normal CSF-T-tau levels (Blennow et al., 1995; Morikawa et al., 1999; Urakami et al., 1999). T-tau therefore has a diagnostic value to discriminate neurodegenerative disorders from pseudodementia due mainly to psychiatric disorders.

4. T-tau and Aβ Combination

The combined evaluation of T-tau and Aβ levels satisfy the criteria for reliable biomarkers described above (The Ronald and Nancy Regan Research Institute of the Alzheimer's Association, 1998). Discrimination of AD from other disorders not associated with pathologic conditions of the brain (CON), other neurologic disorders (ND) and non-AD types of dementia (NAD) was significantly improved by the combined assessment of Aβ42 and tau (Hulstaert et al., 1999). At 85% sensitivity, specificity of the combined test was 86%

(95%CI: 81% to 91%) to discriminate between presence or absence of dementia compared with 55% (95% CI: 47% to 62%) for Aβ42 alone and 65% (95% CI: 58% to 72%) for tau alone. The combined test at 85% sensitivity was 58% (95% CI: 47% to 69%) specific for NAD. Lastly, the combined measure of CSF Aβ42 and tau meets the requirement for clinical use in discriminating AD from normal aging and other neurological disorders (Hulstaert et al., 1999).

5. Hyperphosphorylated Tau Protein (P-Tau)

In AD, numerous phosphorylation sites in the tau protein have been identified. In its hyperphosphorylated state, tau protein looses its ability to stabilize microtubules, causing axonal instability, which contributes to the dysfunction in their transport ability (Ferreira et al., 1989; Iqbal et al., 1997). Moreover, hyperphosphorylated tau promotes tau aggregation and NFT formation (Goedert et al., 1993).

5.1. Hyperphosphorylated T-Tau Levels in CSF

Five different ELISAs have been developed for different phosphorylated epitopes of tau, including threonine 181 and 231 (P-Tau $_{181+231}$) (Blennow et al., 1995), threonine 231 and serine 235 (P-Tau $_{231+235}$) (Ishiguro et al., 1999), serine 199 (P-Tau $_{199}$) (Ishiguro et al., 1999), threonine 231 (P-Tau $_{231}$) (Kohnken et al., 2000) and serine 396 and 404 (P-Tau $_{396+404}$) (Hu et al., 2002). A marked increase of P-tau levels was found in AD patients using these different ELISA methods.

Normal P-tau levels were found in psychiatric disorders such as depression (Buerger et al., 2003) and in chronic neurological disorders such as amyotrophic lateral sclerosis (ALS), Parkinson's disease (Blennow et al., 1995; Sjögren et al., 2002) and other dementias, including VaD, FTD and LBD (Parnetti et al., 2001; Vanmechelen et al., 2000; Hampel et al., 2004). This implies that P-tau is considered to reflect the phosphorylation state of tau, being a more direct biomarker for discriminating AD from others dementias.

Further, after acute stroke, there is a marked increase in CSF T-tau, while CSF P-tau levels do not change (Hesse et al., 2001). These findings suggest that P-tau is not simply a marker of neuronal damage (as T-tau is considered to be), but could specifically reflect the phosphorylation state of tau, and thus possibly the formation of NFTs.

6. CSF Biomarkers in Mild Cognitive Impairment

So far, there is no established method to predict progression to Alzheimer's disease in individuals with MCI. Early studies indicated that CSF biomarkers could be useful for defining a subgroup of patients with MCI at especially high risk of developing AD (Blennow, Hampel, 2003; Hampel et al., 2004; Maruyama et al., 2004).

In MCI cases that deteriorate to AD, high T-tau levels discriminate MCI patients that progress to AD from those that do not progress (Arai et al., 1997). In another study, low Aβ42 and high T-tau levels were found in 90% of the MCI that progressed to AD as compared with the 10% stable MCI (Riemenschneider et al., 2002). In a similar way, a marked increase in P-tau levels was found in MCI, who at follow-up had progressed to AD (Buerger et al., 2002). A combination of CSF T-tau and Aβ42 at baseline yielded a sensitivity of 95% and a specificity of 83% for detection of incipient AD in patients with MCI (Hansson et al., 2006).

These findings suggest that CSF biomarkers may be of use in the clinical identification of AD in the very early phases of the disease and thus facilitate early intervention.

7. Establishment of Reference Values

For the introduction of these assays in clinical practice, adequate reference values are of importance. To date a big study was carried out on CSF T-tau and Aβ42 levels in a large sample (n=231) of individuals without neuronal or psychiatric dysfunctions, with a large age range (21-93 years). Because CSF T-tau levels correlate with age, separate reference intervals have been calculated for different age categories. The reference values for CSF-tau were <300 ng/L in the group having 21-50 years of age, < 450 ng/L in the group of 51-70 years of age and < 500 ng/L in the group of 71-93 years of age. Because there was no correlation between age and CSF-Aβ42 levels and no significant differences were found when the sample was divided into different age groups, only one reference value for CSF-Aβ42 was set (normal levels > 500 ng/L; Sjögren et al., 2001).

Conclusions

Combining data from several studies (Knopman, 2001; Blennow and Hampel, 2003), the specificity for the three CSF biomarkers was 90% or more and the sensitivity was 86% for Aβ42, 81% for T-tau and 80% for P-tau. The combination of the three CSF biomarkers enhances the precision of the AD diagnosis.

In summary, biological marker research is most advanced in the area of AD diagnosis. Attention has been focused on finding one single marker for AD. This seems possible only if the marker is related to a pathogenic step that is unique to AD. However, neural and synaptic degeneration is not only found in AD, but in most chronic degenerative disorders of the brain. Similarly, deposition of Aβ is not specific for AD, but also found in normal aging (Beach, 2008) and LBD (Deramecourt et al., 2006), while formation of PHF into tangles may occur also in normal aging and FTD (Von Bergen et al., 2001). This reduces the likelihood of finding one single biochemical marker for AD. Today, the combined CSF biomarkers, when used as adjuncts to the clinical diagnosis, have the potential to help differentiating AD from normal aging (Castaño et al., 2006), progressive supranuclear palsy (Holmberg et al., 2003), FTD (Grossman et al., 2005), VaD (De Jong et al., 2006) and alcoholic dementia.

Future studies on CSF Aβ42 and T-tau will assist in the characterization of risk indicators by which measure the risk of cognitive decline and dementia for the initiation of earlier intervention and possibly prevention strategies.

Lastly, it is reasonable to assume that the examined CSF markers should not be used as isolated tests and the clinical diagnosis of AD should be based on cumulative information gained from clinical examination (memory disturbance), neuropsychological test batteries, brain-imaging (SPECT, MRI) and CSF biochemical assays. Biomarkers may have their most important value early in the course of the disease when the diagnosis is the most troublesome and may be an aid for clinicians in setting the diagnosis already at the first clinical evaluation.

References

American Psychiatric Association: Diagnostic and Statistical Manual of Mental Disorders, ed4 (DSM-IV). Washington, American Psychiatric Association, 1994.

Andreasen N, Vanmechelen E, Van de Voorde A, Davidsson P, Hesse C, Tarvonen S, et al. Cerebrospinal fluid tau protein as a biochemical marker for Alzheimer's disease: a community-based follow-up study. *J Neurol Neurosurg Psychiatry* 1998; 64: 298-305.

Andreasen N, Sjögren M, Blennow K. CSF markers for Alzheimer's disease: total tau, phospho-tau and Abeta42. *World J Biol Psychiatry* 2003; 4(4): 147-155.

Andreasen N, Vanmechelen E, Van de Voorde A, Davidsson P, Hesse C, Tarvonen S, et al. Cerebrospinal fluid tau protein as a biochemical marker for Alzheimer's disease: a community-based follow-up study. *J Neurol Neurosurg Psychiatry* 1998; 64: 298-305.

Arai H, Nakagawa T, Kosaka Y, Higuchi M, Matsui T, Okamura N, et al. Elevated cerebrospinal fluid tau protein level as a predictor of dementia in memory-impaired patients. *Alzheimer's Res* 1997; 3: 211-213.

Beach TG. Physiologic origins of age-related beta-amyloid deposition. *Neurodegener Dis* 2008; 5(3-4): 143-145.

Blennow K, Hampel H. CSF markers for incipient Alzheimer's disease. *Lancet Neurol* 2003; 2: 605-613.

Blennow K, Wallin A, Agren H, Spenger C, Siegfried J, Vanmechelen E. Tau protein in cerebrospinal fluid: a biochemical diagnostic marker for axonal degeneration in Alzheimer's disease? *Mol Chem Neuropathology* 1995; 45: 788-793.

Buerger K, Zinkowski R, Teipel SJ, Tapiola T, Arai H, Blennow K, et al. Differential diagnosis of Alzheimer's disease with cerebrospinal fluid levels of tau protein phosphorylated at threonine 231. *Arch Neurol* 2002; 59: 1267-1272.

Buerger K, Zinkowski R, Teipel SJ, Arai H, De Bernardis J, Kerman D. Differentiation of geriatric major depression from Alzheimer's disease with CSF tau protein phosphorylated at threonine 231. *Am J Psychiatry* 2003; 160: 376-379.

Castaño EM, Roher AE, Esh CL, Kokjohn TA, Beach T. Comparative proteomics of cerebrospinal fluid in neuropathologically-confirmed

Alzheimer's disease and non-demented elderly subjects. *Neurol Res* 2006; 28(2): 155-163.

De Jong D, Jansen RW, Kremer BP, Verbeek MM. Cerebrospinal fluid amyloid beta42/phosphorylated tau ratio discriminates between Alzheimer's disease and vascular dementia. *J Gerontol A Biol Sci Med Sci* 2006; 61(7): 755-758.

Deramecourt V, Bombois S, Maurage CA, et al. Biochemical staging of synucleinopathy and amyloid deposition in dementia with Lewy bodies. *J Neuropathol Exp Neurol* 2006; 65(3): 278-88.

Ferreira A, Busciglio J, Caceres A. Microtubule formation and neurite growth in cerebellar macroneurons which develop in vitro: evidence for the involvement of the microtubule-associated proteins, MAP-1a, HMW-MAP2 and Tau. *Brian Res Dev Brain Res* 1989; 49(2): 215-228.

Goedert M. Tau protein and the neurofibrillary pathology of Alzheimer's disease. *Trends Neurosci* 1993; 16: 460-465.

Griffin WS. Inflammation and neurodegenerative diseases. *Am J Clin Nutr* 2006; 83(suppl): 470S-474S.

Grossman M, Farmer J, Leight S, Work M, Moore P, et al. Cerebrospinal fluid profile in frontotemporal dementia and Alzheimer's disease. *Ann Neurol* 2005; 57(5): 721-729.

Grundke-Iqbal I, Iqbal K, Tung YC, Quinlan M, Wisniewski HM, Binder LI. Abnormal phosphorylation of the microtubule-associated protein τ (tau) in Alzheimer cytoskeletal pathology. *Proc Natl Acad Sci* 1968; 83: 4913-4917.

Haass C, Schlossmacher MG, Hung AY, Vigo-Pelfrey C, Mellon A, Ostaszewski BL, et al. Amyloid β-peptide is produced by cultured cells during normal metabolism. *Nature* 1992; 359: 322-325.

Hampel H, Buerger K, Zinkowski R, Teipel SJ, Andreasen N, Sjögren M, et al. Measurement of phosphorylated tau epitopes in the differential diagnosis of Alzheimer disease: a comparative cerebrospinal fluid study. *Am J Psychiatry Arch Gen Psychiatry* 2004; 61: 95-102.

Hampel H, Teipel SJ, Fuchsberger T, et al. Value of CSF beta-amyloid 1-42 and tau as predictors of Alzheimer's disease in patients with mild cognitive impairment. *Mol Psychiatry* 2004; 9: 705-710.

Hansson O, Zetterberg H, Buchhave P, Londos E, Blennow K, Minthon L. Association between CSF biomarkers and incipient Alzheimer's disease in patients with mild cognitive impairment: a follow-up study. *Lancet Neurol* 2006; 5: 228-234.

Hasegawa M. Biochemistry and molecular biology of tauopathies. *Neuropathology* 2006; 26: 484-490.

Hesse C, Rosengren L, Vanmechelen E, Vanderstichele H, Jensen C, Davidsson P, et al. Cerebrospinal fluid markers for Alzheimer's disease evaluated after acute ischemic stroke. *J Alzheimer Dis*; 2000; 2: 199-206.

Hesse C, Rosengren L, Andreasen N, Davidsson P, Vanderstichele H, Vanmechelen E, Blennow K. Transient increase in CSF-total-tau but not phospho-tau after acute stroke. *Neurosci Lett* 2001; 297: 187-190.

Holmberg B, Johnels B, Blennow K, Rosengren L. Cerebrospinal fluid Abeta42 is reduced in multiple system atrophy but normal in Parkinson's disease and progressive supranuclear palsy. *Mov Disord* 2003; 18: 186-190.

Hoozemans JJM, Veerhuis R, Rozemuller JM, Eikelenboom P. Neuroinflammation and regeneration in the early stages of Alzheimer's disease pathology. *Int J Neuroscience* 2006; 24: 157-165.

Hu YY, He SS, Wang X, Duan QH, Grundke-Iqbal I, Iqbal K, et al. Levels of nonphosphorylated and phosphorylated tau in cerebrospinal fluid of Alzheimer's disease patients: an ultrasensitive bienzyme-substrate-recycle enzyme-linked immunosorbent assay. *Am J Pathol* 2002; 160: 1269-1278.

Hulstaert F, Blennow K, Ivanoiu A, et al. Improved discrimination of AD patients using [beta]-amyloid$_{(1-42)}$ and tau levels in CSF. *Neurology* 1999; 52(8): 1555-1562.

Iqbal K, Grundke-Iqbal I. Machanism of Alzheimer neurofibrillary degeneration and the formation of tangles. Mol Psychiatry 1997; 2: 178-180.

Ishiguro K, Ohno H, Arai H, Yamaguchi H, Urakami K, Park JM et al. Phosphorylated tau in human cerebrospinal fluid is a diagnostic marker for Alzheimer's disease. *Neurosci Lett* 1999; 270: 91-94.

Kanai M, Matsubara E, Isoe K, el at. Longitudinal study of cerebrospinal fluid levels of tau, Abeta 1-40, and Abeta 1-42(43) in Alzheimer's disease: a study in Japan. *Ann Neurol* 1998; 44: 17-26.

Kanemaru K, Kameda N, Yamanouchi H. Decreased CSF amyloid beta42 and normal tau levels in dementia with Lewy bodies. *Neurology* 2000; 54: 1875-1876.

Kang J, Lemaire HG, Unterbeck A, Salbaum JM, Masters CL,Grzeschik KH, Multhaup G, Beyreuther K, M¨uller-Hill B. The precursor of Alzheimer's disease amyloid A4 protein resembles a cell surface receptor. *Nature* 1987; 325: 733–736.

Knopman DS. Cerebrospinal fluid β-amyloid and tau proteins for the diagnosis of Alzheimer disease. *Arch Neurol* 2001; 58: 349-350.

Kohnken R, Buerger K, Zinkowski R, Miller C, Kerkman D, De Bernardis J et al. Detection of tau phosphorylated at threonine 231 in cerebrospinal fluid of Alzheimer's disease patients. *Neurosci Lett* 2000; 287: 187-190.

Maruyama M, Matsui T, Tanji H, et al. Cerebrospinal fluid tau protein and periventricular white matter lesions in patients with mild cognitive impairment: implications for 2 major pathways. *Arch Neurol* 2004; 61: 716-720.

Masters CL, Simms G, Weinman NA, Multhaup G, McDonald BL, Beyreuther K. Amyloid plaque core protein in Alzheimer's disease and Down syndrome. *Proc Natl Acad Sci* 1985; 82: 4245–4249.

McKhann G, Drachman DA, Folstein MF, Katzman R, Prince D, Stadlan EM: Clinical diagnosis of Alzheimer's disease: Report of the NINCDS-ADRDA work group under the auspices of the Department of Health and Human Services task force on Alzheimer's disease. *Neurology* 1984; 34: 939-944.

Morikawa Y, Arai H, Matsushita S, Kato M, Higuchi S, Miura M, Kawakami H, Higuchi M, Okamura N, Tashiro M, Matsui T, Sasaki H. Cerebrospinal fluid tau protein levels in demented and non-demented alcoholics. *Alcohol Clin Exp Res* 1999; 23: 575-577.

Otto M, Wiltfang J, Tumani H, Zerr I, Lantsch M, Kornhuber J, Weber T, Kretzschmar HA, Poser S. Elevated levels of tau-protein in cerebrospinal fluid of patients with Creutzfeldt- Jacob disease. *Neurosci Lett* 1997; 225: 210-212.

Parnetti L, Lanari A, Amici S, Gallai V, Vanmechelen E, Hulstaert F. CSF phosphorylated tau is a possibile marker for discriminating Alzheimer's disease from dementia with Lewy bodies. Phospho-Tau International Study Group. *Neurol Sci* 2001; 22: 77-78.

Petersen RC. Normal aging, mild cognitive impairment, and early Alzheimer's disease. *Neurologist* 1995; 1: 326-344.

Petersen RC, Parisi JE, Hohnson KA, Waring SC, Smith GE. Neuropathological findings in patients with a mild cognitive impairment. *Neurology* 1997, 48: A102.

Riemenschneider M, Lautenschlager N, Wagenpfeil S, Diehl J, Drzezga A, Kurz A. Cerebrospinal Fluid Tau and β-Amyloid 42 proteins identify Alzheimer Disease in subjects with Mild Cognitive Impairment. *Arch Neurol* 2002; 59: 1729-1734.

Schoonenboom N, Mulder C, Van Kamp J, Mehta S, Scheltens P, Blankstein M, Mehta P. Amyloid β 38, 40 and 42 species in cerebrospinal fluid: more of the same? *Ann Neurol* 2005; 58: 139-142.

Seubert P, Vigo-Pelfrey C, Esch F, Lee M, Dovey H, Davis D, et al. Isolation and quantification of soluble Alzheimer's β-peptide from biological fluids. *Nature* 1992; 359: 325–327.

Sjögren M, Davidsson P, Wallin A, Granerus AK, Grundström E, Askmark H, et al. Decreased CSF β-amyloid42 in Alzheimer's disease and amyotrophic lateral sclerosis may reflect mismetabolism of β-amyloid induced by separate mechanism. *Dement Geriatr Cogn Disord* 2002; 13: 112-118.

Sjögren M, Vanderstichele H, Agren H, et al. Tau and Aβ42 in cerebrospinal fluid from healthy adults 21-93 years of age: establishment of reference values. *Clin Chem* 2001; 47 (10): 1776-1781.

Sjögren M, Minthon L, Davidsson P, Granèrus AK, Clarberg A, Vanderstichele H, et al. CSF levels of tau, β-amyloid 1-42 and GAP-43 in frontotemporal dementia, other types of dementia and normal aging. *J Neural Transm* 2000; 107: 563-579.

St George-Hyslop PH, Tanzi RE, Polinsky RJ, Haines JL, Nee L, Watkins PC, et al. The genetic defect causing familial Alzheimer's disease maps on chromosome 21. *Science* 1987; 235: 885–890.

Storey E, Spurck T, Pickett-Heaps J, et al. The amyloid precursor protein of Alzheimer's disease is found on the surface of static but not activity motile portions of neurites. *Brain Res.* 1996; 735(1): 59-66.

Strozyk D, Blennow K, White LR, Launer LJ. CSF Aβ42 levels correlate with amyloid-neuropathology in a population-based autopsy study. *Neurology* 2003; 60: 652-656.

The Ronald and Nancy Regan Research Institute of the Alzheimer's Association. The National Institute on Aginig Working Group: Consensus report of the Working Group on Molecular and Biochemical Markers of Alzheimer's Disease. *Neurobiol of Aging* 1998; 19: 109-116.

Urakami K, Mori M, Wada K, Kowa H, Takeshima T. Harai H, et al. A comparison of tau protein in cerebrospinal fluid between corticobasal degeneration and progressive supranuclear palsy. *Neurosci Lett* 1999; 259: 127-129.

Vanmechelen E, Vanderstichele H, Davidsson P, Van Kerschaver E, Van Der Perre B, Sjögren M, et al. Quantification of tau phosphorylated at threonine 181 in human cerebrospinal fluid: a sandwich ELISA with a synthetic phosphopeptide for standardization. *Neurosci Lett* 2000; 285: 49-52.

Von Bergen M, Barghom S, Li L, Marx A, et al. Mutations of tau protein in frontotemporal dementia promote aggregation of paired helical filaments by enhancing local beta-structure. *J Biol Chem* 2001; 276(51): 48165-74.

Wiltfang J, Esselmann H, Bibl M, et al. Highly conserved and disease-specific patterns of carboxyterminally truncated Abeta peptides 1-37/38/39 in addition to 1-40/42 in Alzheimer's disease and in patients with chronic neuroinflammation. *J Neurochem* 2002; 81: 481-496.

Yamazaki T, Koo EH, Selkoe DJ. Cell surface amyloid beta-protein precursor colocalizes with beta 1 integrins at substrate contact sites in neural cells. *J Neurosci* 1997; 17(3):1004-1010.

Index

D

E

F

G

guidelines, 45, 48, 54, 143, 150, 155, 161,
168, 199, 205, 206, 217, 230
gyrus, 183, 184, 191, 192, 194, 198

H

HA, 200, 241
half-life, 191
hallucinations, 142, 148
hands, 219
health, x, 44, 137, 138, 139, 145, 147
Health and Human Services, 241
health care, 139
health problems, x, 137, 145
hearing loss, 148, 159
heart failure, 147
hemiparesis, 53
hemispheric asymmetry, 188
hepatic encephalopathy, 147
heterogeneity, 77, 84, 98, 170, 188
heterogeneous, 177, 188, 230, 231
heterozygotes, 220
high risk, 179, 195, 236
high-risk populations, 86
hippocampal, 183, 186, 188, 194, 198, 202,
210, 211, 214, 218, 219, 222, 225, 228
hippocampus, 29, 50, 83, 156, 177, 182,
183, 185, 186, 194, 200, 201, 211, 233
histochemical, 192
histological, 200
history, 45, 57, 100, 140, 144, 146, 159,
192, 195, 198
HIV, 141, 148, 149, 172
homocysteine, 159, 162
homogeneity, 118
homogeneous, 188
hormones, 149
hospitalization, 148
human, 3, 6, 15, 22, 23, 37, 39, 40, 77, 100,
108, 109, 138, 139, 187, 195, 200, 201,
221, 233, 240, 242
human body, 108
human brain, 3, 22, 100, 109, 187, 233
humans, 199
hybrid, 97, 109

hybridization, 8
hydrocephalus, 46, 205
hyperhomocysteinemia, 178
hyperlipidemia, 178
hyperphosphorylation, 177, 206, 230
hypometabolic, 193
hypoperfusion, 189, 196, 198
hypothesis, 3, 20, 28, 30, 34, 49, 56, 148,
159, 177, 195, 209, 221, 232, 234
hypothyroidism, 45, 141

I

iatrogenic, 148
ideal, 48, 180, 184, 185, 200, 204, 230
identification, vii, xi, 1, 2, 34, 88, 119, 121,
133, 158, 162, 175, 176, 177, 182, 205,
228, 236
identity, 17
illumination, 12
image, 12, 14, 50, 92, 130, 194, 216, 219
image analysis, 92, 194, 219
imagery, 26
images, 34, 90, 92, 98, 125, 126, 129, 134,
182, 189, 193, 204
imagination, 40
imaging, xi, 176, 180, 181, 182, 185, 187,
190, 191, 194, 195, 198, 199, 200, 201,
202, 203, 204, 206, 207, 208, 209, 211,
212, 214, 215, 217, 218, 219, 220, 237
imaging modalities, xi, 176
imaging techniques, 185, 201
immobilization, 7, 12
immune system, 15
immunization, 22
immunoprecipitation, 15
immunotherapy, 3, 178
impairments, 36, 46, 202
improvements, 120, 201
in vitro, 209, 239
in vivo, 3, 22, 27, 49, 54, 57, 143, 156, 181,
190, 199, 200, 201, 202, 208, 223
incidence, 177
income, 138
independence, 47, 150, 181, 223

N

O

T